CLINICAL EXAMINATION

A Problem Based Approach

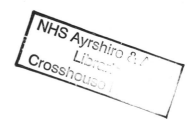

CLINICAL EXAMINATION

A Problem Based Approach

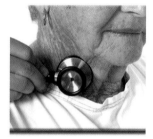
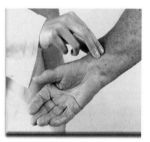

Balakrishnan Kichu R Nair

University of Newcastle & Hunter New England Health, Australia

editor

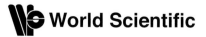

World Scientific

NEW JERSEY · LONDON · SINGAPORE · BEIJING · SHANGHAI · HONG KONG · TAIPEI · CHENNAI

Published by

World Scientific Publishing Co. Pte. Ltd.

5 Toh Tuck Link, Singapore 596224

USA office: 27 Warren Street, Suite 401-402, Hackensack, NJ 07601

UK office: 57 Shelton Street, Covent Garden, London WC2H 9HE

British Library Cataloguing-in-Publication Data
A catalogue record for this book is available from the British Library.

CLINICAL EXAMINATION
A Problem Based Approach

ISBN-13 978-981-4273-91-6
ISBN-10 981-4273-91-0

Typeset by Stallion Press
Email: enquiries@stallionpress.com

Printed in Singapore by Mainland Press Pte Ltd.

To

Usha, Narayani and Gayatri

Preface

Clinical medicine is an art and a science. It is all about taking a history, doing a physical examination, followed by targeted investigations to reach a diagnosis and finally, to chart appropriate management. Unfortunately, the teaching of these skills has taken a back seat in our curricula in the past few decades.

Textbooks and journals cannot replace good patient-oriented teaching. As Osler said "he who studies medicine without books sails an uncharted sea, but he who studies medicine without patients does not go to sea at all". The practice of medicine is all about patient care. In the words of Francis Peabody, "the secret of patient care is caring for the patient". We are here to care for our patients. We should be teaching and learning this everyday with, and from, our patients.

This book is an attempt to revisit good old-fashioned history taking and physical examination. This is more relevant in this century, because of, or in spite of, all the modern technologies. With history and good clinical examination, a working diagnosis can be made in most clinical cases. This book is written by practicing clinicians, all of whom share that philosophy.

We have taken a different approach to a system based examination. Each chapter begins with a patient problem. Some new chapters such as vascular examination and rheumatology have been introduced.

I have to thank the authors for their work, together with Stephen Mears and Kathy Ingham for their editorial support. William Browne was there from the very beginning. My thanks also to the editorial staff at the World Scientific Publishing company, especially Shelley Chow and Jihan Abdat.

I hope the book meets the learners' unmet needs.

Kichu Balakrishnan Nair
Newcastle, Australia, 2010

Foreword
Paul Finucane FRCPI, FRACP

The ability to apply one's medical knowledge and clinical skills to the assessment and management of patients is the essence of competent medical practice. Though it takes most doctors a good many years to move from a level of basic clinical competence to one of mastery, the novice medical student is obliged to go through the painful process of acquiring basic clinical competence in the first place. Most of us doctors have vivid memories of the frustration that we encountered as junior clinical students when the confusion generated by a patient's story was compounded by even more confusing findings on clinical examination. How we marvelled at the ability of senior colleagues to ask the critical questions that we had failed to ask, to reach a provisional diagnosis based on this history, to seek and find the confirmatory signs on clinical examination and to establish the diagnosis in an apparently effortless way. Many of us will also remember the occasion when suddenly, the "lights went on" and for the first time, the presentation of a patient's disease made total sense and correlated with the pathophysiological description contained in the textbooks. It was that "Eureka" moment that convinced many of us that we possibly had what it takes to become a doctor after all.

At the time when I was a novice clinical student, I would have greatly valued having a text which demystified clinical medicine, which clearly described how patients should be examined and which related clinical signs to my rudimentary understanding of the structure and function of the human body. I would have welcomed a text with a user-friendly layout, with clear diagrams and clinical photographs which added clarity and interest to the subject matter. I would have enjoyed references to relevant aspects of medical history. I would have appreciated a book that was rich in aphorisms, pearls of wisdom and humour. In short, I would have valued having access to Professor Kichu Nair's excellent book.

In taking the reader through each of the major body systems, this practical little book is reminiscent of a series of clinical bedside teaching sessions delivered by a number of charismatic and enthusiastic clinical teachers. The frequent presentation of clinical vignettes serves to ground the material in a real clinical context. This helps to link theoretical concepts with clinical practice. The book will help both novice and more senior students to develop and hone their clinical competence.

Professor Paul Finucane FRCPI, FRACP
Foundation Head
Graduate Medical School
University of Limerick, Ireland

Foreword
Elizabeth L Cobbs MD FACP

Across the globe, institutions of medical education are improving the quality of their curriculum, while simultaneously focusing on the importance of patient-centered care. Healthcare has entered a new era and so must the tools that support clinical learning. The dramatic increase of knowledge, treatments and funding involved in healthcare over the last 50 years has presented enormous challenges. At the same time, the growing number of older patients and the typical complexity of their interacting conditions, acute and chronic, require healthcare professionals to achieve high levels of competency in treating older adults. No textbook of adult medicine is complete without special attention to this important and growing demographic imperative. Proficiency at history taking and physical examination remains as the foundation of effective medical practice.

This vibrant and comprehensive text provides the broad, fundamental knowledge and skills necessary to the practice of clinical medicine. Within the pages of this cheerful and engaging book, the authors present concise chapters covering the essentials of history-taking and physical examination in an organ system format. Interspersed throughout are pearls of historical and clinical wisdom to help the learner acquire new information with lasting connections to other knowledge domains. A colorful array of pictures depicting physical findings, radiographs, test reports, and other helpful schematics are plentiful throughout the book. Summary tables present useful information in a taut, easy-to-read format. *Kichu's Thoughts* highlights key bits of clinical wisdom and project the feeling of bedside teaching rounds with an experienced, master clinician.

The importance of communication is a theme that weaves throughout the text and repeatedly reminds us that the patient is the center of our caring and practice. Without the patient as our focus, we are entirely without purpose or place. This theme is particularly germane to clinicians in the practice of caring for older persons, where values and preferences regarding healthcare treatments are as varied as the diverse and heterogenous populations of older persons whom we endeavor to serve. The final chapter is devoted entirely to the examination of the older person and makes this book a true treasure. Along with information about how to effectively conduct an examination of an older adult, learners are gently introduced to the plethora of physical findings that may be normal in later life. The importance of frailty and other geriatric syndromes is introduced, and the format of using a problem-oriented approach offers an efficient and practical method for assessment and treatment planning.

This book offers readers a joyous journey into learning history and physical examination. For experienced clinicians and teachers, this volume will revive us with reminders of the wonders of the human body and spirit. We are indebted to Professor Nair and his authors for a treasure trove of knowledge.

Elizabeth L Cobbs MD FACP
Associate Professor, Medicine and Health Care Sciences
George Washington University
Chief, Geriatrics and Extended Care
Washington DC Veterans Affairs Medical Center
Washington DC, USA

About the Authors

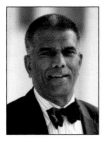

Balakrishnan R Kichu Nair
Professor Balakrishnan R Kichu Nair AM, FRACP, FRCPE, FRCPI, FRCPG is the Clinical Professor of Medicine and Associate Dean of Continuing Professional Development at the School of Medicine and Public Health at the University of Newcastle, Australia. He is the Director of the Medical Professional Development Unit of Hunter New England Health. He is a member of the National Panel of examiners and member of the examination committee of the Royal Australasian College of Physicians. Professor Nair is a Senior Examiner and member of the Board of Examiners of the Australian Medical Council. He received the Order of Australia (AM) for contributions to medical education.

David Abernethy
Dr Abernethy MB ChB, FRACP is a Senior Lecturer in Neurology at the University of Otago, Wellington. He has extensive experience teaching and examining medical students and residents in neurology, and is an examiner for the Royal Australasian College of Physicians.

Shamasunder H Acharya
Dr Acharya MRCP, FRACP is a Consultant Endocrinologist at the John Hunter Hospital, Newcastle, Australia.

William Browne
Dr Browne FRACP, is a Geriatrician, Eastern Health, Melbourne, Australia.

Arvind Deshpande
Dr Deshpande FRCS (Glasgow), FRCS (Edinburgh), FRACS (Vascular), DDU (Vascular), is the Director of Vascular Surgery at John Hunter Hospital and also holds a Conjoint appointment as Senior Clinical Lecturer in Vascular Surgery at The University of Newcastle Medical School, Australia.

Paul Frankish
Dr Frankish FRACP, is the Clinical Leader of Gastroenterology at North Shore Hospital, Auckland, New Zealand. He has previously chaired the committee for examinations of the Royal Australasian College of Physicians in New Zealand and was the senior examiner in adult internal medicine from 2002 to 2006.

Michael Hayes
Dr Michael W Hayes MBBS, FRACP, is a Staff Specialist General Physician trained in Respiratory and Sleep Medicine currently employed as a General Physician in General Medicine at the Calvary Mater Hospital, Waratah. He is also working in the Department of Respiratory and Sleep Medicine at the John Hunter Hospital, Australia.

Scott Kinlay
Dr Kinlay PhD, FRACP, is an Associate Professor in Medicine in Harvard Medical School and the Director of the Cardiac Catheterization Laboratory and Vascular Medicine Service at the VA Boston Healthcare System in Boston, Massachusetts. He is also the Director of Intravascular Ultrasound at the Brigham and Women's Hospital and Co-Director of the Brigham and Women's Hospital & Boston VA Interventional Cardiology Fellowship Training Program. He is a Fellow of the Royal Australasian College of Physicians, Cardiac Society of Australia and New Zealand, American College of Cardiology,

Society of Vascular Medicine and Society for Cardiovascular Angiography and Interventions. He is an Associate Editor of *Circulation* and Editorial Board Member of *Vascular Medicine*.

Michael Lowe

Dr Lowe FRACP, is the Clinical Dean of Flinders University Northern Territory Clinical School in Darwin. He is the co-author of the text book *Ethics and Law for the Health Professions*, published in Australia by Federation Press. His current interests include clinical ethics, medical education, chronic disease, and indigenous health.

Rowan McIlhagger

Dr McIlhagger MBChB, MRCP, graduated from Aberdeen University in 2003 and is currently a Specialty Registrar in Geriatric Medicine in South-East Scotland.

John van der Kallen

Dr van der Kallen MBBS (UNSW), B Med (Sci), FRACP is a practising Rheumatologist in Newcastle, Australia. He currently works in private practice and as a staff specialist at the Royal Newcastle Centre, John Hunter Hospital, Australia. He has had a long history of teaching undergraduate and post-graduate students. His major interests include osteoporosis and inflammatory rheumatological conditions.

Peter Wark

Dr Wark is a Senior Staff Specialist Respiratory Disease and Clinical Associate Professor at the University of Newcastle, Australia. Peter is also Senior Staff Specialist in the Department of Respiratory and Sleep Medicine, John Hunter Hospital, Newcastle, Australia.

Contents

chapter | 1

Histories, Note Taking and Clinical Reasoning

Michael Lowe and Kichu Nair

Introduction

A proficient history and clinical examination are central features of medical practice. Together, the history and examination perform several vital functions. They:

- establish rapport between the clinician and patient,
- establish physical contact between the clinician and patient,
- enable an accurate diagnosis to be made (70–90% of all diagnoses are established by the end of the history and examination),
- identify the severity of symptoms,
- determine prognosis,
- improve efficiency and lower the costs of care (as a consequence of clinicians modifying their pre-test calculation of probability of disease and tailoring subsequent investigations appropriately).

It is therefore important for all doctors to both possess the skills needed to perform a comprehensive history and examination, and be aware of the accuracy (sensitivity, specific and likelihood ratios) and

> **Kichu's thoughts . . .**
>
> Do not say Mr Singh is a poor historian. The historian is the one who documents the history! When you cannot take a detailed history, it is often because the patient is unwell, confused or has speech or communication problems.

precision (degree of agreement between observers) of various aspects of the clinical assessment.

Using an Interpreter

Many interviews with patients will need to be done with the help of interpreters. It is important to realise that many patients who appear to speak English (or any other language) well, may not actually have the capacity to express higher level concepts well. Interpreters are often underused.

At the start of interviews that use interpreters, try to arrange the seating where the interpreter is sitting to the side of the patient. This will allow you to face the patient directly.

When using an interpreter, you should first introduce yourself to both the patient and the interpreter. If the interpreter has not already done so, you should then introduce the interpreter to the patient. The interpreter and the patient need to talk to each other for a short while before the session begins, to establish who the interpreter is in relation to the patient and why they are there.

You should then brief the interpreter on the topic for interpreting, using this opportunity to explain, in plain standard English, any specialised words or concepts that may be difficult to interpret. Not all interpreters have specific health interpreting training.

Tell the interpreter that during the interview, if they are not clear on something that you have said, they should stop you and ask for a more detailed explanation.

Speak as clearly as possible, using plain standard English wherever possible. Do not speak too fast. Speak in short sentences so the interpreter can remember clearly what you have said. After each statement you should wait and allow time for the interpreter and patient to answer.

Try to speak directly to the patient rather than to the interpreter. This may take some practice. At the end of the interview you should spend a few minutes with the interpreter to discuss any language or cultural concerns that may have arisen.

History Taking

If you listen hard enough, the patient will often tell you what is wrong with him or her. (In an exam it is even perfectly allowable to ask the patient their diagnosis!) If you are not listening carefully to what the patient is saying, you may miss vital information.

One important aspect of medical interviewing is that while a clinician must treat the complaints of a patient as possible evidence of a medical problem, he or she should not view what the patient says as definitive with respect to what the problem is, or even whether a problem actually exists. During the interview the clinician swings between identifying with the patient's conversation in a way that is similar to normal social conversation, and in viewing the conversation itself as evidence that must be evaluated separately to what the speaker is trying to say.

When patients come to doctors, they will usually have prepared narratives of their illnesses to present. The aims of such narratives may be very varied — they may be structured in such a way as to give the doctor a careful, systematic understanding of every symptom suffered by the patient, or may be deliberately misleading — such as if the patient is trying desperately to reassure both themselves and the doctor that they do not have a greatly feared illness, for example, cancer. Narratives may be based on patients' cultural understandings of illness, or be aimed at expressing distress rather than at analysing illness. In rare cases, patients may deliberately fabricate a history to obtain narcotics or other drugs.

The doctor's job is to restructure the patient's narrative for the purpose of medicine — this may include interpreting the patient's narrative in ways that are different to how the patient interprets them, picking on features that the patient finds unimportant, or even minimising factors that the patient believes should be the main focus of the interaction.

Student doctors frequently take the words of patients literally (if, for example, they say they have had a "heart attack" or "asthma") when they should instead be thinking about what the patient means by stating this. (For example, a patient who says he/she has asthma may have another cause of breathlessness, and a patient with a "heart attack" may have had a cardiac arrest or suffered a broken heart from a failed romance.)

Some doctors may conduct interviews by firing a series of closed questions at patients. This is efficient in some situations where there are limited responses required (such as the decision about whether to remove a plaster) but it risks making major mistakes in diagnosis, and fails to establish rapport. These faults can be avoided by moving gently from open questions towards closed questions (although there are exceptions to this rule in some styles of interviewing as discussed below).

When doctors record the histories that they take from patients, they generally do it in the following order:

1. Presenting symptoms
2. History of present illness
3. Past medical/surgical history
4. Medications
5. Allergies
6. Smoking, alcohol and illegal drugs
7. Family history
8. Social history (including occupational history), followed by
9. Examination
10. Diagnosis or problem list
11. Further investigations
12. Treatment

As medical students are taught to record histories in this way, many doctors also take histories in this order. Those who use this method tend to open the consultation with some identifying data (name, age, occupation, etc.) and some general rapport-promoting questions and then proceed to ask questions in the order that they will record it.

This style of interviewing has many advantages: it flows naturally, as the patient begins with the problem at hand and then delves back into their past. It also allows doctors to write the history as it is given, and they will not generally need to append or modify their notes, thus saving time. This style of history taking also allows doctors to move from open questions (such as "How are you?" or "Can you tell me what's the matter?") to closed questions (such as "Have you got any allergies?", or "Do you smoke?".)

However, there are also a number of problems with this approach. Firstly, it does not easily adapt to patients with multiple problems. Secondly, there is often a clear logical link between items in the social history, drug history or past medical history and the presenting problem, which are better brought out early in the case rather than inferred by the reader at the end. (For example, if a patient with fevers has lived much of their life in the tropics, or a patient with dyspnoea is a heavy smoker, or another patient with dyspnoea is able to play an entire game of football.) There may also be clues in the medication history that point to further medical problems. (For example, a patient with a long history of dyspnoea might reveal that he or she takes antihypertensives, gout medication and antidepressants, but not give any history of hypertension, gout or depression.)

There are several other ways of taking a history. One approach is to start by asking the patient for a *list* of their problems. (Often this method is used in a long case for the postgraduate examination, when there is a limited time to complete the history and examination.) At this stage of the interview, the doctor does not seek any more information about these problems, but merely seeks to list them, and may have to cut the patient off if they try and explain more about each problem. Once this list is finished, the patient is then asked to list their medications. If any other medical problems are suggested by the medication list, these are checked with the patient, and then added to the original problem list. (For example, a patient on long-term warfarin may not have told you about his/her history of pulmonary embolism three months ago.)

The doctor then asks for detailed information about the patient's current level of functioning and activities — their work, their other activities, how they spend their day, why do they have any limitations, etc. The aim of this part of the consultation is to examine the context in which to understand the patient's problems. The doctor also asks in detail about family history, to see if there are underlying hereditary factors that may expose the patient to an increased risk of disease. Habits such as drug and alcohol use, and allergies are also asked at this time.

Occupational history is also important. A patient with shortness of breath may have been exposed to coal dust or asbestos. If a patient had a funny turn and he is a train driver, it may have major implications in future management.

The doctor only goes back to the patient's problems once he or she has a clear understanding of the context in which these problems should be viewed. The doctor then focuses on each problem in detail, and can link them with underlying social and hereditary factors and with each other with comparative ease.

The advantage of this method is that it tends to be very time-efficient, particularly for patients with multiple problems. The logical cause and effects of problems are explored in an appropriate time frame (i.e. going from the underlying cause to the effect), and little is left out. This method can be adapted easily to oral presentations, by writing each section and problem on a card, and shuffling them at the end to put them in the traditional order (although this should not be allowed to obscure the cause and effect relationships).

The problems with this method are that patients may feel as though they have lost rapport with the doctor in the early stages, where their story is interrupted, but this is usually made up later in the interview by the concentration upon social factors. It may also feel unnatural to the doctor. Doctors must begin with a series of closed questions to make the original problem lists, and only ask open questions later in the interview. In situations where the interview must progress through a translator, it can be difficult to capture the social flavour of interactions, and the first method may be easier.

In clinical practice, it is our experience that few patients have detailed medical histories recorded, apart from those with difficult medical problems. For many patients, the scope of the interview will be much narrower (such as in an orthopaedic clinic where the doctor is merely attempting to see whether the plaster can be removed). In other cases (such as in general practice) a picture of the patient may have been built up over a long time, and each consultation only adds a small amount to the underlying picture.

Sometimes after the history and physical examination, you may have to ask a few closed questions. For example, after you find bilateral ballotable kidneys, you may want to explore a family history of polycystic kidneys, cerebral aneurysms and hypertension to tighten up the diagnostic process. What is important is that doctors need to be flexible in their history taking, and continue to be open to the need for a more thorough history where it is required, and be capable of obtaining such a history.

In general, it is best if doctors can practise a number of different interviewing styles and use them as the circumstance requires. (It is worth noting that a university exam would not be a good time to try out a new method of history taking for the first time!)

Presenting a History

It is customary to start presenting a history with a patient profile (i.e. "Mr Jones is a retired truck driver."). Some presenters attempt to make themselves look a little better by commenting favourably on the patient's demeanour ("Mr Jones is a very pleasant retired truck driver") or by adding colourful information (i.e. "Mr Jones is a very pleasant retired truck driver who is a great fan of Elvis"). Although they may be useful at times, these tactics should be used sparingly, as they may distract the listener.

At the beginning of a history presentation, the listener should be informed about where the presenter is going (i.e. "Mr Jones was admitted with fever, cough and confusion. The story of his illness began...").

When a doctor has an underlying theory about the patient's illness, this should be stated overtly to the listener or the reader, who should not have to infer it themselves. So for example, if a young woman presents with dyspnoea, the doctor should not simply state that the patient does not take contraceptives, and leave the listener to infer that he or she is attempting to rule out causes of pulmonary embolism. A better statement would be "The patient has no risk factors for pulmonary embolism, in particular she does not take contraceptives, has had no long trips recently, and has had no previous or family history of coagulation abnormalities." In this way, questions that refer to certain hypotheses should be explicitly linked to those hypotheses during the presentation.

For many diseases, there are a number of important aspects of history that should be grouped together, rather than scattered throughout the history. For example, if a patient presents with ischaemic heart disease, the risk factors of smoking, family history and hyperlipidaemia should all be dealt together in the history of the presenting illness, rather than in their usual places. (i.e. "The only risk factor that this patient has for ischaemic heart disease is that he smokes 20 cigarettes per day. He does not have any family history, and does not have high cholesterol.") Relevant negative findings may be included within these groups of findings. Laboratory data may also be sometimes included briefly in the history of presenting illness or past medical history if it is necessary to understand the story in a logical way.

Medical students are usually directed to ask a wide range of general questions about body systems as part of a systems review. While these should be recorded in the notes, they should not be repeated in verbal presentations. If a relevant positive or negative finding comes up in a systems review, it should be included in the past medical history or history of present illness. An important key to making oral presentations is to know what to include and what to leave out.

If you have placed a piece of social or other history into a part of the history where it does not normally get covered (such as smoking history in the presenting symptom of weight loss and haemoptysis), you should not repeat it later. The aim of the presentation is to briefly but thoroughly explore a patient's problems, not to slavishly follow protocols for discussion.

It should be noted that it is possible to be overly narrative in a presentation. ("First the patient went to doctor A who said this, then he/she went to Dr B who said that, then he/she went back to doctor A, etc.") Remember that a medical history is a particular type of narrative that aims to show cause and effect in order to make sense of the story, not necessarily to render a historically accurate account of a person's business.

Presenting the Examination Findings

At the end of an examination, doctors are expected to present their findings in a logical, systematic way. They are also expected to present a diagnosis if possible and to lay out the course of action that should follow from the findings that they have observed.

> **Kichu's thoughts . . .**
>
> If you hear hoofbeats outside, it is more likely to be from a horse than a zebra. But to make medicine more interesting, it is occasionally a zebra, not a horse!

There are a number of ways that findings can be presented. In an assessment situation, where everyone is highly stressed, it is probably best to report the findings in the sequence in which they were discovered. This way nothing important will be forgotten. After this, the doctor should briefly summarise the important points, give a diagnosis, and possibly a differential diagnosis, and then report where they would go to next. When doctors are summarising their findings, they should not re-state everything again. A summary should summarise (i.e. stick to one or two sentences)!

Making a Diagnosis

The medical history attempts to create a narrative, in which a number of symptoms and signs are placed into a structure of cause and effect. Most fictional stories have an introduction, a temporal sequence and a conclusion. The same is true of medical histories, although this is not always how patients present their stories to the doctor. The doctor attempts to place patient's symptoms into a story that is coherent, and which may then suggest a number of possible theories about what is wrong with the patient.

In general, doctors pick their theories about what is wrong with their patients using several principles that sometimes conflict with one other.

The first principle is that attempts to explain signs and symptoms should follow a logical time sequence. For this reason, the timing of all symptoms should be pinned down as clearly as possible. For example, if a patient presents with diarrhoea, and is known to be on antibiotics, the diagnosis cannot be completely explained by antibiotic-associated diarrhoea if it is known that the diarrhoea was present before the antibiotics commenced.

A second principle is that doctors should attempt to explain the signs and symptoms by starting with common diseases and only move on to less common diseases if things cannot be explained with a common disease. A number of old sayings in medicine involving zebras and other exotic animals attest to the usefulness of this principle. For example, a patient who presents with overweight and abdominal striae is more likely to suffer from plain obesity than from Cushing's disease. (However, it may also be important to rule out Cushing's disease as explained below.) An important limitation of this principle arises from the fact that rare diseases will never be found unless they are looked for, thus doctors must keep their minds open to the possibility of rare diseases, while concentrating upon the probability of common diseases.

A third principle is known as "Ockham's razor". Ockham's razor states that one should not multiply causes unnecessarily. In other words, a simple explanation is more likely to be correct than a complex one. Doctors will therefore first attempt to explain patients' symptoms by using a single disease. If this is not convincing they may attempt to explain it with a number of related conditions, and finally with a number of unrelated conditions. For example, if a young man presents with haemoptysis and haematuria, the doctor may think either of Goodpasture's syndrome (a single disease that explains both symptoms), or Ig A nephropathy with a respiratory infection (diseases which together will cause the clinical picture), or simultaneous chest and urinary infections (unrelated diseases that together will cause the syndrome.) Ockham's razor would suggest that Goodpasture's syndrome would be the first disease to rule out.

A fourth principle that is commonly used by doctors, is that if a diagnosis has severe implications, it should be included as a possibility in order to rule it out. For example, a patient who presents with atypical chest pain will generally need further investigations to rule out ischaemic heart disease, even if the chest pain seems unlikely to be ischaemic in origin, because the consequences of missing a diagnosis of ischaemic heart disease may be serious.

> **Kichu's thoughts . . .**
>
> A young person with multiple organ involvement may have multisystem disease, whereas older patients may often have multiple diseases of multiple systems. Ockham's razor is often not applicable to older patients!

It is also possible to use more quantitative approaches to diagnosis. Such approaches form the basis of a number of computerised diagnostic algorithms which are becoming more commonly used in medicine. Many of these algorithms are based upon Bayes' theorem. Diagnosis using Bayes' theorem begins with the clinician estimating the pre-test probability of the patient having a particular disease. This would be usually estimated by the underlying epidemiology of the disease and the clinical picture of the patient. This probability is then expressed as the odds that the patient will have the disease.

Test results (or even the results of clinical examinations) can then be put in the form of "odds ratios", which in turn can be combined with the pre-test likelihood of a disease, to make a more accurate estimate of the odds that a patient has a disease (the post-test odds). Post-test odds are then converted into post-test probabilities of the disease.

For example, if I believe that a patient has a pre-test probability of having a pulmonary embolism of 20%, this can be translated as odds of 1:4. A strongly positive VQ scan has an odds ratio of close to 7, which can be multiplied by the pre-test odds to give a post-test odds of 7:4 or 63%.

How to Communicate Effectively in the Chart

The Purpose of Medical Records

The primary purpose of medical records is as the note-taker's record of the encounter. Notes should therefore include both factual data and a record of the intellectual process that the author went through so that he or she can refer to this at a later date. Secondary purposes for medical records include for communication with other team members, and for medico-legal purposes, for quality assurance activities and for later audit and research. What is written in the medical notes may eventually impact on resourcing, planning and healthcare research.

In order for medical records to fulfil these purposes, it is essential that they are legible. Anyone who writes in the record must be certain that the following points are clearly identified:

- Patient ID (name, date of birth, HRN)
- Your identity (rank or unit)
- Date and time
- Purpose of record (e.g. "Ward round" or "Asked to see patient re breathlessness")
- Source of information (e.g. patient, relative)
- It is often useful to list the hospital day, the post-op day or the duration of antibiotics
- Signature

The Format of Medical Records

There is no standardised way to write in the notes. Different methods of note taking are required for admission notes, progress notes, discharge summaries and outpatient records. In the future, hospital records are likely to become increasingly computerised, so it is important that the techniques used for writing notes can be adapted to this. (Notes are already computerised in many practices and hospitals.)

The main approaches to note writing that are used are variations on the "Patient-Oriented Medical Record" and "SOAP" as described by Weed in 1968/1969. Weed's method of note taking depends upon making a numbered problem list for each patient, and then addressing each active problem in the notes each day. The problems are each addressed under the headings Subjective, Objective, Analysis, Plan (SOAP). Weed also recommended the use of a flow chart for recording pathology results.

Most physicians today use modified versions of Weed's method. The most common modification is to use a problem list followed or preceded by a narrative. Unlike Weed's approach, the problem lists are rarely formally numbered or addressed by number in the notes. Most medical units include problem lists in the admission notes. Some physicians prefer the list to be written separately on a page at the front of the patients' notes.

Problem lists need to balance conciseness and thoroughness (e.g. if "urinary tract infection" is seen as one problem, "leukocytes in urine", "fever", and "dysuria" should not be listed as additional problems).

Each of the problems is addressed daily on the ward round. If a problem is no longer important, the list can either be re-written, or a dated note made on the original problem list informing that this problem is now resolved.

Many residents also find that the SOAP acronym a useful way of organising their daily notes. This can either be done as Weed intended — with a new SOAP written for each problem, or with a single set of headings that address all the problems.

Flow charts of pathology results are frequently used in ICU, renal wards and other highly technical areas. There is an increasing tendency to not document results obtained from the computer, which is risky both legally and from the point-of-view of efficient decision-making. Important results from the computer should be written in the progress notes to document that the team has discussed them. The team's interpretation of these results should also be noted. Flow charts of results should probably be used more commonly.

The Language of Medical Records

The language of medical records must be respectful of the patient. You should not use disrespectful descriptions of the patient or their condition (such as "gomer" or "acopia"), no matter how amusing these might be. These look very bad when read out in court! Similarly, you should not use abbreviations that are not easily understood or universally acknowledged. RDH (Royal Darwin Hospital) is an example.

You should avoid criticism of other care-givers in the notes. This might otherwise lead to legal action. Short, simple sentences are best (e.g. "Mr Jones is breathless at rest."). Headings and dot points are encouraged. Medical teams find it useful if the medical notes stand out from the other notes (although this can often be inferred from the quality of the handwriting). Leaving some space before and after the medical notes helps with this. There is an extremely limited role for the use of different coloured pens and other such tricks.

Direct quotes are often useful (e.g. "Patient says that 'He would rather die than go to a nursing home.'"). When dealing with a difficult patient or family, write down what was said (e.g. "In the family meeting we advised then that the patient was unlikely to return home but would need nursing home placement."). It is often useful to read the notes back to the rest of the team at the end of the consultation.

The Content of Medical Records

Medical records should include both the objective findings and the thoughts of the team (e.g. you should not write just "LVF" or just "JVP elevated". Both should be combined "Elevated JVP — likely LVF.") Where possible, observations should be quantified (e.g. "He is tachypnoeic rate 24."). When abnormal laboratory results are seen, they should usually be commented on, e.g. "Creatinine is rising (today 224) likely due to gentamicin."

Wherever possible, you should explain the team's thinking in the chart. If it is not apparent to the note-taker, he or she should ask for clarification, e.g. "Mr Jones' confusion is likely to be due to a combination of sepsis and underlying dementia" or "Anaemia noted: If it continues tomorrow we will transfuse." (This is particularly important because many notes are reviewed for evidence of mistakes of management as part of quality assurance activities. If it is not clear why changes to management are made, it is difficult to assess whether the changes were appropriate.)

It is sometimes useful to communicate with other disciplines in the notes (e.g. "Question for surgeons: When do you intend to remove NG tube?" or "Question for physio: Shouldn't this man have a frame rather than a stick?").

Legal Issues

From a legal perspective, the main value of medical records is that they provide a record of happenings. They will therefore be preferred over most verbal testimony if the two are in conflict. Medical records that are incomplete, or those that appear unreliable (i.e. if they appear to have been amended), or records written after the event, are all less valuable. In addition to the suggestions above, legal sources suggest that you should, where possible:

- write notes yourself and sign them;
- never sign an entry on behalf of another staff member;
- do not edit the notations, even for legibility;
- if errors occur, cross out the inaccuracies and initial and date them with a margin note explaining the reason for the change;
- take great care when transcribing treatment orders or reports from an original order or report.

Medical records contain information that is a private matter between the patient and the treating team. Medical students and doctors have sometimes been observed looking up the records of friends and family members who are currently patients. This is entirely unacceptable, unless both patient and treatment team have consented.

Medical records are referred to frequently throughout the day's work. They should not be removed from the ward, and if they are taken to a private area on the ward, the ward clerk should be aware in case they are required.

There are many legal requirements concerning the privacy of medical information. There is not enough space in the current document to detail these, but students need to be familiar with them.

chapter 2

Respiratory Examination

Peter Wark and Michael Hayes

Summary of the Respiratory Examination

General inspection

- Expose the upper body.
- Sit the patient at 45°.

Respiration

- Count the respiratory rate and note if the breathing pattern is abnormal as in Cheyne–Stokes respiration.
- How hard is the patient working to breathe? Note distress and use of accessory muscles.

Cough

- Note the presence of cough.
- Is it productive?
- Is there a sputum container nearby?

Oxygen

- Is the patient on oxygen?
- Is it via mask or prongs?
- What is the flow rate?

Is the patient febrile?

> **Kichu's thoughts . . .**
>
> To say something is normal takes lots of experience.
>
> Practise on percussing and auscultating yourself or on your friends. To put yourself in the patients' position, feel the tracheal deviation yourself and see what is the optimal pressure you should use.

Hands and peripheries

• Check the hands for clubbing, cyanosis and nicotine staining.

Pulses and oxygen saturation

• Take the pulse, note the presence of tachycardia and especially atrial fibrillation.
• If able, record oxygen saturation using an oximeter.

Head/Mouth

• Inspect the face for evidence of central cyanosis, assess for conjunctival pallor.
• The mouth should be examined for the condition of the dentition and gums.

Neck — JVP assessment

• The jugular venous pressure (JVP) should be assessed. It is elevated in congestive cardiac failure, which may be the cause of breathlessness. But it is also elevated in pulmonary hypertension.
• Examine the sub-mental and cervical lymph node chains systematically. Conclude with examining both supraclavicular fossae.

Chest

• Examine the anterior and posterior chest sequentially.

Inspection

• Consider the shape of the chest wall, its movements with respiration and evidence of previous surgery.

Palpate

• Feel for the position of the trachea.
• Assess chest expansion. Is it symmetrical?
• Palpate both axillae for lymph nodes or masses.
• Palpate for vocal fremitus, comparing side to side starting at the apices (including the supraclavicular spaces and axillae when examining anteriorly) and then down the chest.

Percussion

- Percuss the chest from side to side starting at the apices (including the supraclavicular spaces and axillae when examining anteriorly) and then down the chest.
- Compare the percussion note side to side.
- If there is altered percussion, describe the area.

Auscultation

- Auscultate with the diaphragm.
- Auscultate carefully, listening at each place for at least two breaths through the respiratory cycle.
- Start at the supraclavicular fossae and work down, comparing side to side. Remember to listen in both axillae.
- Are the breath sounds normal (vesicular)?
- Are the breath sounds of normal intensity?
- Is there an area of bronchial breathing? If so, accurately describe it.
- Are there added sounds? Describe wheeze, crackles, stridor or a pleural rub. Do these sounds occur throughout the respiratory cycle, are they confined to inspiration or expiration?
- Auscultate for vocal resonance, listening again from right to left, side to side.

Request the patient to perform a forced expiratory time. Alternatively, get him/her to perform spirometry. Review the chest radiograph.

Detailed Respiratory Examination

The phrase "practice makes perfect" may sound trite but it is, in fact, reality with regard to physical examination. Refine your technique by examining numerous "normal" chests and you will appreciate signs of disease far more readily.

Preparing the Patient

It is important to prepare the patient for the examination that will allow you to perform this professionally and efficiently. Remember that the patient's comfort and dignity should be foremost in your mind and that you should always demonstrate this to them and where appropriate, to your examiners. For respiratory patients who may be breathless, minimise their effort and ensure they have access to supplemental oxygen if they need it.

Spend time making the patient comfortable. Ideally they should be undressed to the waist but be attentive to modesty. We find it easiest to begin the examination with the patient lying at 45° to examine the periphery and anterior chest.

Then assist the patient into a sitting position and examine for lymphadenopathy and the posterior chest. Finally, the patient is returned to the original position and further signs (such as the position of the cardiac apex or signs of cor pulmonale) are pursued as needed.

General Observation

Much information can be gleaned from a good hard look at the patient. You should have a mental checklist of questions and a systematised survey as there is a lot of information to be gathered.

What is the general appearance? Are they well or unwell, cachectic from malignancy or severe chronic obstructive pulmonary disease (COPD), or are they obese?

Observe the respiration. Carefully count the respiratory rate. A normal rate is 12 to 16 breaths per minute. Tachypnoea may occur as a result of breathlessness or secondary to a metabolic acidosis. Is the respiratory rhythm abnormal? For example, Cheyne–Stokes respiration is associated with cardiac failure.

How hard are they working to breathe? Increased work of breathing is an important prognostic sign in both acute and chronic respiratory conditions and is closely related to the perception of dyspnoea. Look to see if the patient is using accessory respiratory muscles, such as the sternocleidomastoids and platysma muscles of the neck. Use of these muscles may be particularly prominent in those with severe airflow obstruction and hyperinflation of the chest.

Intercostal recession of the lower chest is also suggestive of hyperinflation as, in this state, the diaphragm is away from the chest wall thus exposing the lower intercostal regions to intrathoracic instead of intra-abdominal pressures.

CASE STUDY 2.1

Joan is a 68-year-old lady with no history of cardiac or respiratory disease. She presents to the emergency room with 24 hours of fever, rigors, cough and breathlessness.

What clinical findings will aid in the diagnosis?
General inspection: Joan is breathless at rest, with obvious distress and tachypnoea.
Hands and peripheries: The presence of clubbing would be unexpected and may indicate an underlying lung malignancy.
Pulses: You would expect tachycardia at rest and assess saturations with oximetry.
Head/Mouth: Assess for conjunctival pallor; undiagnosed anaemia could account also for worsened exertional dyspnoea in COPD.
Neck — JVP assessment: The JVP should be assessed.
Chest inspection: If breathless, look for use of accessory muscles.
Percussion: Percussion is reduced posteriorly in the left chest, compared to the right, though not stoney dull. No difference anteriorly.
Auscultation: Auscultate with the diaphragm. Are the breath sounds of normal intensity? Breath sounds were generally reduced throughout the left lung posteriorly, though more reduced at the left base. Are there added sounds? Coarse crackles were heard throughout inspiration and expiration, throughout the left lung posteriorly. In addition, there was an area of bronchial breathing present at the left base. Vocal resonance on auscultation is increased in the left lung posteriorly.

These findings are consistent with consolidation involving the left lung, at least the left lower lobe. Given the fever and presentation, pneumonia is likely. The reliability of eliciting chest signs in pneumonia has been assessed in comparison to chest radiography (Wipf *et al.*, 1999). The investigators found that the presence of abnormal chest signs in determining pneumonia had a sensitivity of 47–69% and a specificity of 58–75%. The findings with the best agreement between examiners were the presence of crackles in the upright position, reduced percussion note, followed by bronchial breath sounds (Wipf *et al.*, 1999). Joan went on to have a chest radiograph.

(*Continued*)

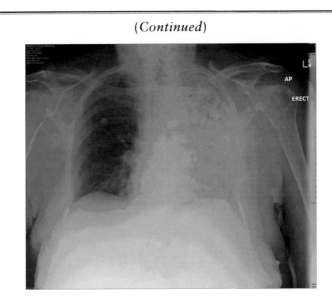

The chest radiograph shows consolidation, predominately involving both the left upper and lower lobes. There is also some volume loss in the left lower lobe suggesting collapse. The left hemidiaphragm is still visble and in keeping with our clinical findings there does not appear to be a pleural effusion.

Note if the patient has a cough and whether they cough during the examination. Determine if the cough is productive of sputum or non-productive. Ask the patient to cough a few times. Note whether the cough is dry or loose and productive. Is it strong and effective or weak and ineffectual? A hoarse voice and a "bovine cough" are suggestive of vocal cord paralysis.

If there is a sputum container available or the patient is able to expectorate, get them to do so. A dry cough may be associated with interstitial lung disease such as pulmonary fibrosis. A productive cough is usually seen with airway inflammation or bronchitis. This can be acute infective bronchitis or may be chronic as is seen in COPD, which is associated with mucus hypersecretion and will lead to cough often with clear mucus (see Fig. 2.1).

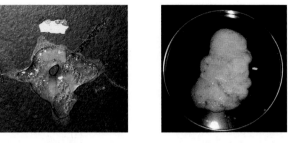

Panel A   **Panel B**

Figure 2.1. Expectorated sputum.

Infection and airway infiltration with neutrophils often leads to the sputum becoming purulent, adopting a green or yellow colour (Fig. 2.1). As mentioned, this may be acute or due to chronic infection as occurs in COPD.

Purulent sputum indicates the presence of neutrophils and the release of their contents during degranulation, especially myeloperoxidase. This is not always indicative of bacterial infection and may occur with inflammation alone, in the case of asthma or during viral infection. In the case of COPD however, the development of more sputum which changes colour and becomes purulent usually indicates a bacterial infection and requires treatment with antibiotics (Anthonisen *et al.*, 1987).

Chronic cough with large volumes of purulent mucus may indicate the presence of bronchiectasis. Acutely, cough and sputum production is also seen with pneumonia, and may also result in haemoptysis or the expectoration of blood. Large volumes of sputum, especially with poor taste, may be indicative of a lung abscess.

Acute breathlessness and haemoptysis may be seen with pulmonary embolus. Lung malignancy may also lead to increased cough and mucus and at times, haemoptysis. Such a development in a smoker or former smoker always requires further investigation. Cardiac failure may also be associated with frothy clear or blood stained mucus.

In Fig. 2.1, Panel A represents a mucus plug which is clear or slightly mucoid in appearance. Panel B is a purulent mucus plug, typical of that seen in acute or chronic bronchitis.

Hands and Peripheries

"Begin with the hands." Nicotine staining denotes use of cigarettes. Pallor may indicate anaemia as the cause of dyspnoea.

Peripheral cyanosis, the presence of a bluish discolouration of the fingers or hands, is due to a high percentage of deoxyhaemoglobin. It is not a reliable sign as it depends upon not only adequate saturation of haemoglobin during transit through the lung but also adequate perfusion of the peripheries.

Clubbing (see Fig. 2.2) can be associated with many respiratory diseases including cystic fibrosis, bronchiectasis, bronchogenic carcinoma or idiopathic pulmonary fibrosis (Table 2.1). Early stages of clubbing may be subtle.

The profile angle and phalangeal depth ratio can be used as quantitative indices to assist in identifying clubbing (see Fig. 2.3). These values rarely exceed 180° and 1.05 respectively in normal subjects.

Head and Mouth

Look for central cyanosis, a blue tinge around the lips associated with deoxygenated haemoglobin. Expose the conjunctiva to look for pallor.

Inspect the oral cavity. Candidiasis may indicate immunosuppression or use of inhaled corticosteroids. Inspect dentition because

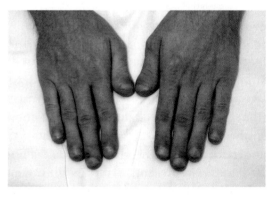

Figure 2.2.   Clubbing.

Table 2.1.   Causes of clubbing.

Respiratory

Primary lung cancer, 35% (non-small cell)

Mesothelioma

Chronic suppurative lung disease (bronchiectasis, cystic fibrosis, empyema, lung abscess)

Idiopathic pulmonary fibrosis (present in 50% of cases)

Cardiac

Cyanotic congenital heart disease

Subacute bacterial endocarditis

Atrial myxoma

Gastrointestinal

Hepatic cirrhosis (hepatopulmonary syndrome), especially primary biliary cirrhosis

Inflammatory bowel disease (both Crohn's and ulcerative colitis)

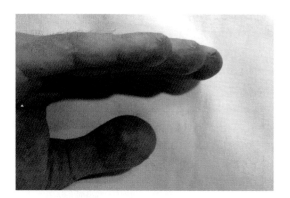

Figure 2.3.   Clubbing — side view.

dental caries and gingivitis are associated with anaerobic chest infections and the development of lung abscess.

The face may reveal evidence of other diseases associated with respiratory complications, including connective tissue diseases such as scleroderma and systemic lupus erythematosis and their associated features.

Neck and JVP

The JVP should be estimated in all patients during the respiratory exam. As described in the cardiovascular chapter (Chapter 3), the patient should be positioned at 45°. While the JVP may be elevated as a consequence of cardiac failure, respiratory diseases are important causes of an elevated JVP too. Right sided heart failure may develop as a consequence of chronic respiratory diseases, especially COPD. This is termed "corpulmonale" and is associated with elevated JVP and peripheral oedema. It may be the sole clinical finding in chronic pulmonary hypertension and may also develop acutely with pulmonary embolus.

It is also important to examine systematically the submandibular, cervical and supraclavicular lymph node chains. These are shown in Fig. 2.4. Feel each of these. Note the size and texture of the node. Lymph nodes increase in size in response to infection or when they are infiltrated by tumour. Generally, they are small and difficult to feel. Small cervical nodes are often present, probably as a consequence of recent or recurring upper respiratory tract infections. These nodes should be smooth with a rubbery texture.

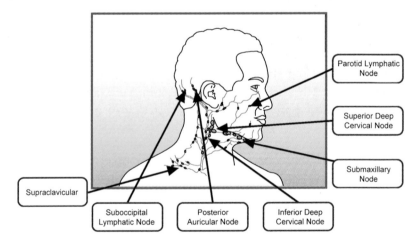

Figure 2.4.   Cervical and supraclavicular lymph node chains.

Malignancy leads to enlarged nodes. Often, they are hard and may be fixed to underlying structures. Lymphoma will often lead to multiple enlarged nodes that may not be hard. Usually there is involvement of other lymph node chains and if you suspect this, always examine for epitrochlear nodes and the abdomen for hepatosplenomegaly. Intrathoracic tumours may spread to the supraclavicular fossae. Involvement of the cervical chain is usually seen with cancers of the head and neck.

Occasionally, nodes may become infected — they then become tender, reddened and warm. This may occur with mycobacterial infections, such as tuberculosis, atypical mycobacteria and while not seen in the developed world, infection with *Mycobacteria bovis* (scrofula). These nodes may even rupture and drain pus. Previous mycobacterial infection can also lead to scarred hard nodes.

Also be aware of the effects of previous radiotherapy and surgery that may lead to an area of scarred hard tissue, especially in the supraclavicular fossa. Finally, examine each of the axillae for lymph nodes. Intrathoracic malignancies again may drain here and metastasise.

Inspection of the Chest

Take time to assess the shape and symmetry of the thoracic cavity. Significant hyperinflation is a feature of severe COPD and may result in an increased anteroposterior diameter of the chest or "barrel chest". This is best appreciated by observing the patient from above whilst they are sitting. The AP diameter will often approach the lateral diameter. While a useful sign if it is present, a barrel chest is only present in 10% of patients with severe airflow obstruction and its absence does not exclude severe airflow obstruction.

Restrictive chest wall disease may arise from distortion of the spine, ribs or sternum. Kyphosis and scoliosis are common especially in the elderly. Asymmetry may also result from any process resulting in loss of lung volume, from lobar collapse to pneumonectomy. In the past, radical surgery was performed for patients with tuberculosis, this approach involved procedures that lead to pleural scarring and lung collapse, the result of which led to dramatic alteration of

CASE STUDY 2.2

David is a 74-year-old man who comes to see you, concerned with a persisting cough and breathlessness on exertion. David is an ex-smoker, he stopped five years ago following coronary stenting for angina, but has a 40 pack-year history of smoking. His breathlessness and cough have worsened since he had the "flu" some three months ago. He is breathless walking on the flat and finds he has to stop and rest every 100 m. The cough is productive of clear sputum, mostly in the morning.

What is the diagnosis?
COPD should be foremost in your mind given David's age and smoking history. Asthma is differentiated from COPD by the presence of reversible airflow obstruction on spirometry; and while this can develop in adults, it is less likely given David's age and smoking history. Important differential diagnoses however, would be exertional angina or left ventricular failure. Other lung disease such as an interstitial lung disease or a pleural effusion is possible.

What clinical findings will aid in the diagnosis?
General inspection: David complains of exertional dyspnoea and is unlikely to be breathless at rest or tachypnoeic.
Hands and peripheries: The presence of clubbing would be unexpected and may indicate a lung malignancy.
Pulses: You would not expect tachycardia at rest, though an irregular pulse may indicate atrial fibrillation and account for exertional dyspnoea.
Head/Mouth: Assess for conjunctival pallor, undiagnosed anaemia could also account for worsened exertional dyspnoea in COPD.
Neck — JVP assessment: The JVP should be assessed. Examine the sub-mental and cervical lymph node chains systematically. Conclude with examining both supraclavicular fossae.
Chest inspection: If David has COPD you may look to see if he is barrel chested. However, this is not likely unless he has severe airflow obstruction.

(Continued)

Percussion: Percussion should be performed in the context of COPD. You will try and determine if the chest is hyperresonant to percussion reflecting hyperinflation of the lungs due to gas trapping. This is a difficult sign to discern and is most likely to be present in those with severe lung disease. Its presence however, is highly specific. In detecting moderate COPD, it has a sensitivity of 32% and specificity of 94% (Badgett *et al.*, 1993).

Auscultation: Auscultate with the diaphragm. Are the breath sounds of normal intensity? David has a reduced intensity of breath sounds bilaterally. This is probably the sign with the best sensitivity to detect moderate COPD. It has a sensitivity of 65% and specificity of 94%, it is also less subjective than hyperresonance on percussion with better interobserver agreement (Badgett *et al.*, 1993). Are there added sounds? There is wheeze heard at both bases posteriorly. The presence of wheeze during tidal breathing in this clinical context would be highly predictive of obstructive airways disease (Straus *et al.*, 2000). However, wheeze is a less sensitive sign in this group than reduced intensity of breath sounds. Wheeze was found to have a sensitivity of 9%, but a specificity of 100% (Badgett *et al.*, 1993).

Other: Request the patient to perform a forced expiratory time. Alternatively, get him to perform spirometry.

The history and physical examination findings already would be enough to make a diagnosis of COPD likely. The pulmonary function tests therefore is not likely to add to your assessment. Spirometry however, would allow you to confirm the diagnosis, determine the severity of airflow obstruction and also assess acute reversibility to short-acting beta agonists.

The spirometry shows severe airflow obstruction with an FEV1 only 21% of the predicted value. The FVC is also reduced to a greater extent than expected and could indicate an element of restriction as well. The chest radiograph shows hyperinflation and a paucity of peripheral lung markings, which are findings consistent with gas trapping and emphysema. The heart is not enlarged and the lung fields are otherwise clear.

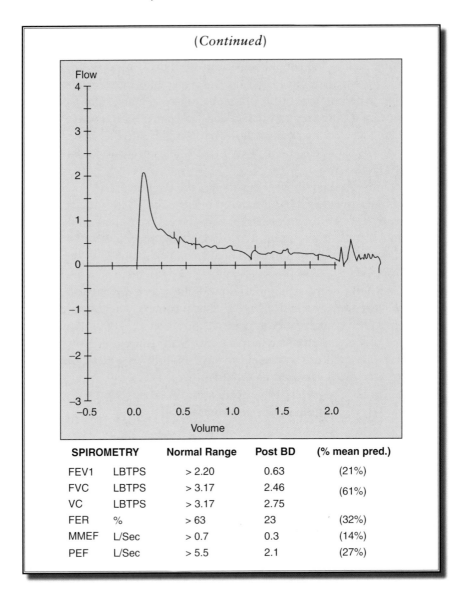

(*Continued*)

SPIROMETRY		Normal Range	Post BD	(% mean pred.)
FEV1	LBTPS	> 2.20	0.63	(21%)
FVC	LBTPS	> 3.17	2.46	(61%)
VC	LBTPS	> 3.17	2.75	
FER	%	> 63	23	(32%)
MMEF	L/Sec	> 0.7	0.3	(14%)
PEF	L/Sec	> 5.5	2.1	(27%)

shape to the thoracic cavity. Over many years, this may result in marked deformity which may lead to severe physiological restriction and progressive respiratory failure. Similar problems may develop with chronic neuromuscular disease associated with wasting of the chest wall musculature.

Note the muscle bulk, as marked wasting may suggest a neuro-pathic or myopathic process that may lead to weakness of the muscles of respiration. Are there any surgical scars from thoracotomy, thoracoscopy or intercostal catheter insertion?

Palpation

Tracheal deviation is a reliable clinical sign when properly performed. To assess its position, ask patient to face straightforward and relax the neck musculature. Place a single finger in the suprasternal notch and gently push forward until the cartilaginous trachea is felt. Gently feel to either side of the cylindrical structure and estimate its position relative to the middle of the supraclavicular notch. This can be uncomfortable for the patient so clearly explain why you are doing this and be as gentle as possible. Perform it on yourself to gauge how firmly you can palpate before causing discomfort.

A trachea deviated from the midline has either been pushed or pulled by a significant anatomical abnormality, usually in the lung apices or mediastinum. The trachea will be pushed away from a large pneumothorax or mass and will be drawn towards collapse or fibrosis. Surgical resection of a lobe or more of a lung (notice thoracotomy scars) will often result in deviation. Occasionally, distortion of the chest wall by severe kyphoscoliosis can result in apparent deviation without underlying parenchymal disease.

A reasonable estimate of the degree and symmetry of thoracic cage excursion can be made. When examining the posterior chest, place a hand with fingers extended on either side of the thorax in a lower lateral position. Point your thumbs towards the midline and try to keep them raised off the skin and steady. Ask the patient to breathe in deeply. Get a general sense of how much the hands and thumbs move away from each other and whether one side moves more than the other. Try to begin with the tips of your thumbs reasonably close to the midline as this makes it easier to see asymmetry of movement.

Palpating for vocal or tactile fremitus remains part of the traditional examination; however, it has limited clinical utility. Its reported kappa value is 0.01, which indicates very poor interobserver agreement (Spiteri *et al.*, 1988).

Percussion

Percussion note can reveal a great deal of information regarding the thoracic cavity, but to be proficient in it requires time and experience. The sensation on percussion felt through the finger tips is as important as the sound.

A cavity that contains air has a deeply resonant sound and feel, whereas solid tissue or fluid will be dull. Percuss the chest from side to side starting at the apices (including the supraclavicular spaces and axillae when examining anteriorly) and then down the chest. Compare the percussion note side to side but make sure you are choosing points equidistant from the midline. Particularly on the posterior chest wall the note will differ slightly at different distances from the midline.

Various disease processes will result in a dull percussion note, including pleural thickening or effusion, consolidation of the underlying lung or masses adjacent to the chest wall.

Hyperresonance on percussion can be found in subjects with severe airflow obstruction. It is a more sensitive sign of hyperinflation than is the presence of a barrel chest. However, being confident that a chest is hyperresonant requires experience and confidence, the presence of loss of cardiac and liver dullness is probably a good clue to reinforce this impression.

Auscultation

Auscultation is widely performed but its interpretation in chest diseases is amongst the most difficult and subjective of assessments; once again, there is no substitute from gaining experience in listening to chests both in disease and health.

Using the diaphragm of your stethoscope, auscultate over the anterior chest, again moving side to side for comparison and starting at the apices. At each position, listen to at least one or two complete respiratory cycles.

Breath sounds from certain lobes of the lung are best heard in different areas and if the examination is not thorough then changes may be missed. The right lung is divided into three lobes: the upper, middle and lower lobes. The left is divided into two, the upper and lower lobes. The left upper lobe further divides into anterior and lingual segments. How the surface anatomy corresponds to lobes is described in Fig. 2.5.

Processes that involve the upper lobes are best heard over the anterior chest with the patient lying at 45°. Involvement of the right middle lobe may only lead to changes heard in the right axilla. Similarly, involvement of the lingula may lead to changes in the left axilla. Transmission of air through the lower lobes is best heard posteriorly. A suggested approach to listening to the chest is given in Fig. 2.5; commence in the area labelled 1, then proceed by numbers, as you will see moving from side to side.

Normal lung sounds are described as vesicular. They arise from turbulent flow of air in the larger airways. Airflow in the smaller airways and alveoli is laminar and produces little noise. Aerated normal lung tissue filters out the high pitched component of the turbulence and thus what you hear at the chest wall are low pitched sounds with no pause between inspiration and expiration. With

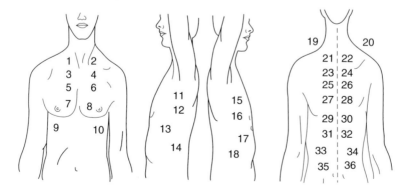

Figure 2.5.   Chest auscultation positions.

experience, one is able to get a feel of how "loud" or "intense" these normal breath sounds are, given the fact that they will vary with the depth of respiration and in relation to the proximity of the stethoscope to large airways.

Causes of Reduced Intensity of Breath Sounds

1. Loss of lung tissue to transmit the sounds. This occurs in emphysema, especially when large bullae are present.
2. Pneumothorax, as the air layer is a barrier to the transmission of sound.
3. Pleural disease such as effusion, thickening or mass, which act as acoustic insulation.

Bronchial Breath Sounds

Bronchial breathing describes an alteration in the quality of the breath sounds. They occur when the lung underlying the area being auscultated is consolidated but the large airways are still patent. The lung now no longer filters out the high pitched sounds, so the breath sounds have a harsher, more blowing quality with some hissing on expiration (like Darth Vader's breathing). Generally there is also a discernable pause between inspiration and expiration.

Added Sounds

Wheeze is a polyphonic musical sound during expiration. It is produced from the vibrating walls of narrowed airways, most commonly from narrowed smaller airways with disrupted laminar flow. Abnormal narrowing of small airways occurs in asthma and pulmonary oedema and is also a dynamic process in COPD.

The presence of wheeze has been described as the most precise indicator of airflow obstruction, if heard without forced expiration (Holleman *et al.*, 1993). However, wheeze is not specific for obstructive airways and other investigators have highlighted these concerns suggesting that it is not appropriate to rely upon a single physical examination finding such as wheeze for a diagnosis (Straus *et al.*, 2000). The value of wheeze to diagnose obstructive airways disease increased in the context of age greater than 45 years, history of smoking or a history of previous obstructive lung disease (Straus *et al.*, 2000). Therefore, spirometry is the test of choice to diagnose obstructive airways disease such as asthma and COPD.

Secretions or sputum in airways, as occurs in bronchiectasis, can also generate a wheeze. An endobronchial foreign body or mass may sometimes produce a wheeze but this will be monophonic as it is localised to a single airway.

Stridor is a harsh inspiratory noise resulting from narrowing of the trachea or larynx. Its presence indicates severe limitation to inspiratory airflow and in an acute setting may indicate a medical emergency.

Crackles are heard when collapsed distal airways or alveoli open rapidly during inspiration. They occur in several pathological processes. The important characteristics to note are the quality and the timing of the crackles.

Coarse crackles that are pan-inspiratory or late inspiratory occur when there is fluid in the small airways and alveoli. This fluid can be an exudate as with infection, a transudate as with pulmonary oedema or blood as with pulmonary haemorrhage. Occasionally, inspiratory and expiratory gurgling can be heard in patients with bronchiectasis. Fine, late inspiratory crackles may be a feature of pulmonary fibrosis.

Pleural friction rub is appreciated as a creaking or groaning sound somewhat akin to a heavy door that needs its hinges oiled. Normally the two layers of pleura slide easily over each other during respiration. When inflamed they become rough and tacky, and grip each other. This may produce a rubbing sound during inspiration and expiration. The pleura may become inflamed with pneumonia, pulmonary infarction from emboli or possibly malignant involvement.

Vocal Resonance

Auscultating for vocal resonance should be done in the same areas as described above. Traditionally this is done by getting the patient to repeat the number "99". Changes to vocal resonance occur through changes in the conduction of air through the lung. Where there is a pleural effusion, with fluid between the lung and chest wall or in the case of a pneumothorax where there is air, vocal resonance is markedly reduced. Where the lung is collapsed and little or no air conducted, vocal resonance is reduced. In the case of consolidation, vocal resonance is usually reduced. However, in cases often where bronchial breathing is present, the quality of speech while reduced may become clearer, this is described as whispering petriloquy.

Table 2.2. Clinical signs of consolidation, collapse, pleural effusion and pneumothorax.

	Consolidation	Collapse	Pleural effusion	Pneumothorax
Trachea	Usually unchanged	Shifted toward collapse, may not be detectable if lower lobes are involved	Shifted away, often no change if accumulates slowly	Shifted away
Percussion	Reduced	Reduced	Stony dull	Hyperresonant
Intensity breath sounds	Reduced	Reduced, may be absent	Very reduced or absent	Reduced
Added breath sounds	• Coarse crackles common • Bronchial breath sounds may be present	• Coarse crackles may occur • Fixed wheeze may be heard if a proximal airway is narrowed	May be coarse crackles, even bronchial breathing above the effusion	Absent

Forced Expiratory Time (FET)

Forced Expiratory Time is a manoeuvre where the patient is asked to sit upright, to maximally inhale and then to exhale through an open mouth as forcefully as possible. The clinician listens over the trachea in the suprasternal notch.

Obstructive airways disease is associated with a longer expiratory time, up to 20 seconds. Expiration time of greater than nine seconds was highly predictive of airflow obstruction (FEV1/FVC < 70%). Taken together with wheeze during tidal breathing, prolonged FET of more than nine seconds is highly predictive of airflow obstruction. In subjects over 60 years, using the FET manoeuvre with a cutoff value of six seconds will correctly diagnose the greatest number of subjects with obstructive airways disease (Schapira *et al.*, 1993).

If able however, perform spirometry. Spirometry is the timed measurement of dynamic lung volumes during forced expiration and inspiration to quantify how effectively and how quickly the lungs can be emptied and filled (Fig. 2.6). The measurements usually made are the vital capacity (forced and/or unforced), forced expiratory volume in one second and the ratio of these two volumes (FEV1/FVC).

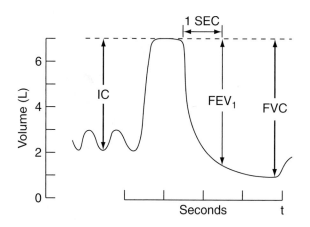

Figure 2.6. Spirometry expiratory volume time curve (adapted with permission from Pierce *et al.* (2005)).

Correctly performed, spirometry is the most valuable tool to quickly assess lung function and is necessary to make the diagnosis of obstructive and restrictive lung disease.

Figure 2.6 is an example of a spirometry volume/time curve. It measures expiratory flow in the first one second, FEV_1 and the forced vital capacity, FVC.

A full description of spirometry and its interpretation is beyond the scope of this book but readers are referred to Pierce *et al.* for their excellent and concise description (Pierce *et al.*, 2005).

CASE STUDY 2.3

Richard is a 54-year-old man, who has noticed that he has become more breathless gradually over the last six weeks. He has developed a dry cough. He is a smoker, but has no history of cardiac or respiratory disease.

What clinical findings will aid in the diagnosis?
General inspection: Richard is not breathless at rest, but is with minimal exertion.
Hands and peripheries: Clubbing is present.
Pulses: 90/minute, regular.
Head/Mouth: Assess for conjunctival pallor central cyanosis.
Neck — JVP assessment: The JVP should be assessed. May also look for distended superior vena caval veins that occur with obstruction due to malignancy.
Chest: Percussion is reduced posteriorly mid way up the left chest, and at the base it is stony dull.
Auscultation: Are the breath sounds of normal intensity? Breath sounds are reduced throughout the left lung posteriorly. Are there added sounds? A few coarse inspiratory crackles are heard mid-way up the posterior left lung. Vocal resonance is reduced from mid way down the posterior left lung.

These findings are consistent with a left sided pleural effusion, while the presence of clubbing in this context makes a primary lung malignancy the most likely diagnosis.

(Continued)

It is important to be able to differentiate between the presence of consolidation and pleural fluid. A summary of the clinical findings that should help do this are described in Table 2.2. Richard went on to have a chest radiograph. This confirmed the presence of a left sided pleural effusion with some associated consolidation above the effusion. The fluid was drained and cytology confirmed the presence of an adenocarcinoma.

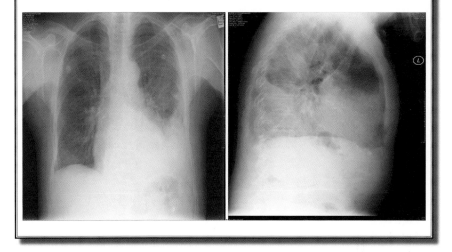

References

1. Anthonisen NR, Manfreda J, Warren CP *et al*. Antibiotic therapy in exacerbations of chronic obstructive pulmonary disease. *Ann Intern Med* 1987; 106(2): 196–204.
2. Badgett RG, Tanaka DJ, Hunk DK *et al*. Can moderate chronic obstructive pulmonary disease be diagnosed by historical and physical findings alone? *Am J Med* 1993; 94(2): 188–196.
3. Holleman DR, Simel DL, Goldberg JS. Diagnosis of obstructive airways disease from the clinical examination. *J Gen Intern Med* 1993; 8: 63–68.
4. Pierce RJ, Hillman DR, Young IH *et al*. Respiratory function tests and their application. *Respirol* 2005; 10: S1–S10.

5. Schapira RM, Schapira MM, Funahashi A *et al.* The value of the forced expiratory time in the physical diagnosis of obstructive airways disease. *JAMA* 1993; 270(6): 731–736.
6. Spiteri MA, Cook DG, Clark SW. Reliability of eliciting physical signs in examination of the chest. *Lancet* 1988; 1: 873–875.
7. Straus SE, McAlister FA, Sackett DL *et al.* The accuracy of patient history, wheezing, and laryngeal measurements in diagnosing obstructive airway disease. *JAMA* 2000; 283(14): 1853–1857.
8. Wipf JE, Lipsky BA, Hirschmann JV *et al.* Diagnosing pneumonia by physical examination: Relevant or relic? *Arch Intern Med* 1999; 159(10): 1082–1087.

chapter | 3

Cardiovascular Examination

Kichu Nair, Scott Kinlay and William Browne

Cardiovascular Examination

Examination of the cardiovascular system is an important part of the assessment of almost every patient. In the vignette described in Case Study 3.1, you are face to face with a patient whose history strongly suggests a cardiac problem. Physical examination will help with the rapid assessment that this patient so urgently needs.

Kichu's thoughts . . .

When confronted with a seriously ill patient, history, examination and investigation may all need to take place at once — but a high degree of thoroughness is always required. Always come back later to complete the history and examination. There are no short-cuts in medicine!

CASE STUDY 3.1

A Man with Chest Pain and Breathlessness

A 65-year-old man presents to the emergency department with breathlessness and chest pain for the last 30 minutes. He has a history of diabetes and hypertension. The pain is central and radiates to his left arm. He appears sweaty, pale and anxious.

What is the differential diagnosis for this presentation and what signs on examination will help to distinguish these?

Summary of Cardiovascular Examination

- **History taking**
  This is where the most important information is communicated! The history will guide most of what you do next. The history above (Case 3.1) will raise immediate concern about a serious cardiac problem. Measurement of the so-called vital signs — the pulse rate, blood pressure and estimation of arterial oxygen saturations as well as an ECG should be performed while the clinician proceeds with a focused history and examination.
- **Position the patient**
  The patient should be positioned in a bed propped up at 45 degrees.
- **Expose the patient**
  The patient should have their chest and lower legs exposed. If the patient is a female, she could have a folded towel placed over her breasts.
- **Lighting and comfort**
  Lighting should be placed so it goes slightly obliquely across the patient's chest and neck. This will allow the apex beat and JVP to be seen more easily.
- **General inspection**
  This stage of the examination begins immediately and continues indefinitely during all time spent with the patient. Is the patient distressed, anxious, pale, flushed or relaxed and well? If, while you are observing the patient, you assess for pedal oedema, this will save some time and give you a good hint for later JVP estimation.
- **Hands and peripheries**
  Many valuable signs can be found in the hands and peripheries, and quickly identified. Check the hands for clubbing, cyanosis and, where appropriate, signs of endocarditis.
- **Pulses**
  Palpate the pulses in the hands, and centrally — either brachial or carotid pulses. Do not rely on automated pulse measurement

which can be unreliable in the setting of atrial fibrillation, low cardiac output states and a number of other conditions.

- **Blood pressure assessment**
  Check this by palpation and auscultation. Usually brachial measurement is sufficient but pressures in the lower limbs are occasionally useful. Postural blood pressure changes are very common in older patients and should form part of any comprehensive cardiovascular examination.

- **Head/mouth**
  Inspect the face for evidence of central cyanosis, malar flush and evidence of endocarditis (in the appropriate context). The mouth should be examined for the condition of the dentition as well as evidence of the high arched palate of Marfan's syndrome.

- **Neck — JVP assessment**
  The JVP is an important guide to pressure in the right atrium. It is elevated in conditions such as congestive cardiac failure, tricuspid regurgitation and pulmonary hypertension and its height should be estimated in every patient. In Case 3.1 or 3.2, its elevation would suggest cardiac failure. A skilled observer can also obtain useful information from the waveform of the JVP.

- **Examine the chest**

  Inspection:
  Consider the shape of the chest wall, its movements with respiration, and evidence of previous surgery, such as sternotomy or the presence of a cardiac pacemaker or defibrillator. Inspect for the position of the apex beat.

  Palpate apex:
  Feel for the position of the apex beat using the flat portion of the fingers applied gently to the precordium. Rolling the patient to the left can be helpful in some patients to identify the apex position (but not to localise).

- **Auscultation of the heart**
  Auscultate with the bell and diaphragm. (Cardiac ausculation in Case 3.1 might reveal an S3 in the presence of cardiac failure or an S4, which can be heard in some patients with acute myocardial infarction.)

- **Examine the legs and sacrum**
  The presence of oedema suggests cardiac failure (there are other causes!). Sometimes pedal oedema can be looked for at the time of general inspection, but sacral oedema must always be checked for at this stage.
- **Examine the abdomen**
  Palpate the abdomen for evidence of ascites, a pulsatile liver, both of which can be features of advanced congestive cardiac failure.

Note: In a focused clinical examination (such as in primary care or a follow-up appointment), only part of this examination would be performed.

Positioning and Exposing the Patient

Take a few moments to prepare the patient for physical examination. Ensure the patient is as comfortable as possible. Even in the acutely unwell patient such as those in Cases 3.1 and 3.2, positioning the patient correctly allows an efficient and accurate examination.

Ideally the patients should be sitting at a 45-degree angle in a bed. Patients should have their chest, arms and legs exposed. Cover the breasts of female patients with a towel or loose piece of clothing.

CASE STUDY 3.2

Harry

A 60-year-old farmer presents to a rural hospital with a six-week history of fever and fatigue. He had rheumatic fever as a child but has been well since. He has lost 10 kg since becoming unwell. He looks sweaty and unwell. His pulse is 100 beats per minute and regular. His blood pressure is 145/70. He has a temperature of 38°C. His oxygen saturation on pulse oximetry is 96%. His fingers appear clubbed and there a splinter haemorrhage in the nail bed if his left index finger. His JVP is not elevated. He has subconjunctival pallor and both a retinal and subconjuntival haemorrhages of his right eye. His apex beat is undisplaced and he has a loud systolic murmur at the apex of his heart

> ### (*Continued*)
>
> radiating to his axilla. Abdominal examination reveals a palpable spleen. He has a blacked area on his right great toe with normal peripheral pulses.
>
> *What diagnosis best fits this constellation of history and findings? What other signs might be present?*

Lighting and Comfort

Lighting should allow the assessment of skin colour and the contour of the neck. Lighting should be placed so it goes slightly obliquely across the patient's chest and neck. This will allow the apex beat and JVP to be seen more easily.

Where possible, try to ensure a quiet environment (rare in hospitals).

General Inspection

Take a few moments to look at the patient's face, level of distress, use of accessory muscles of respiration, any abnormal pulsations in the chest and neck, and whether they look unwell.

Occasionally a relevant diagnosis may be suggested by the patient's general appearance, such as hypo- or hyperthyroidism, acromegaly, or other conditions such as Marfan's syndrome, Down's syndrome or Turner's syndrome — conditions that may be associated with cardiovascular complications. What is the patient's habitus? Is he or she obese? Does the patient appear cachectic — an emaciated state that denotes serious illness, including severe cardiac failure, malignancy, or malnutrition. Sometimes, a spot diagnosis may be made even at this early stage of proceedings, but this should not detract the examiner from completing an exam that will establish potential complications of the diagnosis.

Hands and Peripheries

Valuable information can be found long before beginning the direct examination of the heart.

- **Clubbing**
  Clubbing refers to swelling of the terminal phalanges due to oedema and dilation of capillaries and arterioles. The finding was described by Hippocrates in the presence of empyema.

Causes of clubbing	
Cardiac	Endocarditis
	Cyanotic congenital heart disease
	Conditions causing right to left shunt
Respiratory	
(Refer to Chapter 2)	Neoplasms
	Pulmonary fibrosis
Gastrointestinal	Suppurative lung disease
Idiopathic	Cirrhosis
	Inflammatory bowel disease

It is detected as a change in the angle between the nail bed and the base of the finger. Usually this angle is less than 180 degrees, but in clubbing the angle is equal to or greater than 180 degrees. In addition to the change in the angle of the nail bed, the nail bed itself becomes quite spongy. The nail can feel as if it floats on the underlying tissue. This finding is associated with bacterial endocarditis and with congenital cyanotic heart disease. There are many other causes.

- **Peripheral cyanosis**
  Peripheral cyanosis is a blue discolouration of the fingers or extremities caused by the presence of deoxyhaemoglobin in the subepidermal blood vessels of the peripheries. When seen in the presence of central cyanosis, this reflects systemic hypoxia. However, it is commonly due to poor peripheral perfusion as can

be seen in low cardiac output states, Raynaud's phenomenon, poor arterial flow and impaired venous return.

Stigmata of Endocarditis

Look for the following signs in the hands or feet:

- **Osler's nodes**
  These are tender subcutaneous nodules seen in the finger palps or the thenar eminences. These can be erythematous, haemorrhagic, macular or papular.
- **Janeway lesions**
  These are non-tender, erythematous, haemorrhagic, or pustular lesions, often on the palms or soles.

  Effectively the only difference between these two stigmata of endocarditis is that Osler's nodes are painful whereas Janeway lesions are not, although Janeway's original description makes no mention of this. Both have been found to be due to septic emboli in some cases, and to sterile vasculitis in others. The distinction is therefore an artificial one and has no particular diagnostic significance.
- **Splinter haemorrhages**
  These are thin black streaks under the finger nails. They are most often traumatic and caused by splinters! They are a common physical finding in bacterial endocarditis caused by small haemorrhages in the capillaries of the nail bed.

Other Peripheral Signs of Cardiovascular Disease

- **Xanthomata**
  These are caused by localised deposits of cholesterol and other lipid material within the dermis. They are yellow in colour and have a firm, rubbery texture similar to that of a rheumatoid nodule. There are a number of forms of xanthomata, some of which are relatively specific for particular subtypes of dyslipidaemia.

Tuberous xanthomata are relatively large xanthomata that appear especially at flexural areas. They can come and go over a period of weeks depending on fluctuations in serum lipid levels. They can be seen in any form of hyperlipidaemia.

Eruptive xanthomata are small inflammatory lesions that occur in crops and are associated with any form of hyperlipidaemia. When due to the hypertriglyceridaemia of diabetes, they are called xanthoma diabeticorum.

Tendon xanthomas are seen principally in patients with type II hyperlipidaemia, rarely in type III. They are xanthomas found over tendons, commonly the Achilles tendon and the extensor tendons of the hand.

Palmar xanthomas are small, bead-like xanthomas found over the palmer creases in about half of patients with type III hyperlipidaemia.

- **Central cyanosis**
Central cyanosis reflects systemic hypoxia. It may be seen in patients with congenital cyanotic heart disease or acute hypoxia from pulmonary oedema.

- **Malar flush**
This is a blue/red flush of the cheeks that is classically associated with mitral stenosis but which is also seen in some patients with significant pulmonary hypertension and reduced cardiac output due to other causes, more commonly in people who are outdoors in the sun.

> **Kichu's thoughts . . .**
>
> All signs are in conjunction with other signs.
>
> A patient with a malar flush and splinter haemorrhages may be an avid gardener if you see him working in the backyard; but not if he is febrile, looks unwell and is in hospital.

- **Xanthelasma**
These are pale yellow eruptions seen in the periorbital skin and inner eyelids. They are associated with types II and III hyperlipidaemia, but they can also be seen in some people without abnormal lipid metabolism.

- **Jaundice**
  Patients may develop jaundice in the presence of haemolysis due to a prosthetic heart valve, or from turbulent flow associated with endocarditis.
- **Subconjunctival haemorrhages**
  These are seen in cases of bacterial endocarditis.
- **Ear lobe creases**
  Ear lobe creases have been associated with coronary artery disease. However, the sensitivity and specificity of this correlation is not high.

Fundoscopy

The fundus is the only part of the body where the microvasculature can be directly visualised at the bed side. A description of some important signs visible on fundoscopy can be found in Chapter 5 on neurological examination. Findings pertinent to the cardiovascular exam are included below.

Roth spots may be observed in the fundus of patients with endocarditis. These are small white centred retinal haemorrhages, the white centre being due to fibrin deposition.

You could see arterial pulsations in aortic regurgitation; so aortic incompetence can be diagnosed by fundoscopy even before you listen to the heart!

Note that the normal pulsations seen in the fundus are seen in the veins, not the arteries, because as each arterial pulse brings more blood into the closed space of the eye, the only substance that can make space for it in the eye is the venous blood.

Hypertension affects the microvascular arteries.

Hypertensive retinopathy is graded in the following manner:
Grade 1: "Silver wiring" of the retinal arteries due to sclerosis of the vessel wall.
Grade 2: Arterioles indent the veins where they cross (arteriovenous nipping), as well as silver wiring as above.

Grade 3: Flame-shaped haemorrhages, soft exudates (cotton wool spots caused by localised tissue ischaemia) or hard exudates (caused by lipid accumulation), as well as silver wiring and arteriovenous nipping.
Grade 4: Same as Grade 3 but with the presence of papilloedema.

Pulses

Pulse characteristics are often assessed at the radial and carotid arteries. However, all of the peripheral pulses should be examined. Palpation of both radial pulses simultaneously and a radial and femoral pulse together will help establish the presence of obstructive disease in the more proximal segments of the arterial tree.

The initial assessment of pulse rate, volume and character is usually obtained from the radial pulse. The radial pulse is typically on the radial side of the palmer aspect of the wrist, about two centimetres proximal to the thenar eminence. The pulse is gently gripped with the index finger on the palmer side of the wrist and the thumb on the dorsum of the wrist. The pulse is felt with the wrist flexed and pronated. The brachial pulse is on the medial and anterior part of the elbow crease. The femoral pulse can be palpated below the inguinal ligament. Be sure to explain to the patient what you are doing before attempting to palpate the femoral pulse! (Did you know the dominant artery in the hand is the ulnar artery? Even so, the ulnar pulse may be difficult to find.)

The timing of the pulse at the wrist should happen simultaneously with the timing of the pulse in the femoral artery. If the femoral pulse occurs significantly later than the radial pulse, then this is known as radiofemoral delay. Radiofemoral delay is classically attributed to coarctation of the aorta, usually due to narrowing of the aorta just beyond the origin of the left subclavian branch. It is more often seen in young men. Sometimes a noticeably lower pulse volume in the femoral artery compared to radial artery is all that is appreciated rather than the classic delay in the femoral pulse.

In older patients, radiofemoral delay can potentially occur due to differences in peripheral artery calcification and stiffness between the

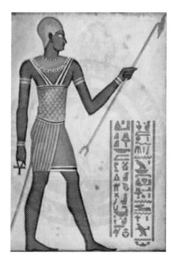

Historical Aside: The Pulse in Ancient Medicine

". . . Examining is like one counting a certain quantity with a bushel, or counting something with the fingers . . like measuring the ailment of a man in order to know the action of the heart." Quoted from the Edwin Smith Papyrus

The ancient Egyptions were known to measure the pulse as part of medical examination, possibly as early as 3000 BC.

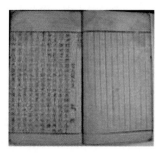

The Chinese wrote numerous books on the technique of pulse taking and its interpretation. The *Mai jing* ("The Pulse Classic"), a massive ten-volume treatise, was a compilation of all of the knowledge on the pulse and describes in detail the correct method for the examination of the pulse.

lower limbs and upper limbs arteries. Typically stiffer arteries lead to an increase in pulse wave velocity with more rapid propagation of the pulse wave. These patients also tend to have hypertension.

Coarctation is sometimes diagnosed in older adults and should not be dismissed because of older age (although advanced atherosclerosis or arteriosclerosis may be a more common cause in the elderly.)

Pulse Rate

The emergence of automatic blood pressure and heart rate measurement by machine has tended to diminish the practice of manually estimating heart rate. However, machines can be wrong, particularly with arrhythmia, and a manual assessment should assess the accuracy of any machine reading.

Count the number of beats per minute. It is often convenient to count the number of beats over 15 seconds and then multiply by four. However, if the pulse is slow or irregular counting over a full 60 seconds will be more accurate. A normal resting heart rate ranges between 60 and 100 beats per minute. Highly trained athletes may have heart rates well below this range. A slow pulse (less than 60 bpm) is termed bradycardia. A fast heart rate (greater than 100 bpm) is termed tachycardia.

It is normal for the pulse rate to vary slightly with respiration, particularly in the young. This is called sinus arrhythmia, and is related to differential filling of the left and right side of the heart, and changes in vagal tone with inspiration and expiration. Typically the heart rate increases slightly during inspiration, and decreases with expiration. As it is partly mediated by vagal tone, this effect, like vagal tone, tends to decline with age. If unsure, ask the patient to hold their breath and see whether the pulse is regular.

When taking a pulse, do not press too hard or you may feel your own pulse.

Rhythm of the Pulse

The pulse is regular with sinus rhythm (apart from the caveat of sinus arrhythmia described above). A very rapid regular rhythm may indicate sinus, supraventricular or ventricular tachycardia. An irregular pulse can be regularly irregular (a recurring pattern such as bigeminy or type II heart block) or irregularly irregular (no clear pattern, such as atrial fibrillation).

Volume of the Pulse

The volume of the pulse is best assessed by palpating one of the larger arteries such as the carotid, brachial or femoral pulses. It is a subtle sign that requires experience over many years and many patients for the examiner to recognise low and high volume pulses. Some examiners prefer to use the thumb to palpate carotid and brachial pulses. A semi-quantitative scale is used to describe pulse volume (increased, normal, reduced, absent).

Character of the Pulse

This refers to an impression of the pulse waveform derived during palpation. Again, like volume, it needs to be examined at one of the large arteries.

Some abnormalities of pulse are described below.

- **Anacrotic (or slow-rising) pulse**
  This is seen in aortic stenosis, and refers to a pulse wave that is slow rising with generally flat volume associated with a low cardiac output and prolonged left ventricular ejection time. It suggests more severe aortic stenosis.
- **Bisferiens pulse**
  This is a more difficult pattern to recognise and is best palpated over the carotid arteries. It is characterised by two systolic peaks and is seen in aortic regurgitation with or without aortic stenosis, and in some patients with hypertrophic cardiomyopathy.
- **Diacrotic pulse**
  This is also a pulse with two peaks — one in systole and the other in early diastole. It may be seen after the administration of nitrates in otherwise normal subjects, in febrile patients or in cardiac

tamponade, congestive cardiac failure or shock, where a ventricular contraction delivers a small volume of blood into a non-rigid arterial circulation.

- **Plateau pulse**
  A slow rising pulse with a flattened peak. This is seen in severe aortic stenosis cases.
- **Collapsing pulse**
  This is a sign of aortic regurgitation, although it is sometimes also seen in patients with a hyperdynamic circulation and with a rigid arterial system. A stiff arterial system leads to an accentuated systolic peak in the peripheral pulses. The pulse has an early peak and then quickly falls away, giving it a tapping quality. The preferred method is to palpate the brachial pulse with the whole palm applied to the flexor aspect of the wrist, and then elevate the patient's wrist. This accentuates the tapping quality of the pulse. (Your colleagues will be impressed with your clinical skills!) The collapsing pulse is also referred to as Corrigans or a water-hammer pulse, after a 19th-century toy that was a vacuum tube containing water or mercury that was flipped creating a tapping or hammer sensation at the finger tips (a most arcane term — perhaps the Game-Boy rumble would be more recognisable today).

  When a collapsing pulse is detected, look for the following signs (although these are rarely seen in societies where advanced bacterial endocarditis is rare or where advanced cardiac imaging is performed for the mildest form of valvular abnormalities).

  There are a number of other signs that can be found in aortic regurgitation. These are usually only done once the condition is already confirmed, and are probably more used for demonstrating aspects of the disease rather than for diagnosis.

  - *Duroziez's sign*
    This is seen in severe aortic regurgitation. Place the diaphragm of the stethoscope over the femoral artery and press downwards. Initially a systolic murmur will be heard. Gradually increase pressure over the artery; a diastolic murmur will

become evident also related to the flow reversal with profound aortic regurgitation. Now tilt the proximal edge of the stethoscope further downwards — if aortic regurgitation is present, the systolic murmur is accentuated and the diastolic component is diminished. Now tilt the distal edge of the stethoscope downwards, the diastolic component will now be accentuated and the systolic reduced ("D for distal and diastolic!") This sign has a positive predictive value of close to 100% for aortic regurgitation, and can detect this lesion in some patients in whom it is not possible to hear the characteristic diastolic murmur on auscultation of the heart (e.g. acute aortic regurgitation due to acute bacterial endocarditis).

○ *Traube's sign*
   A "pistol shot" sound heard over the femoral artery with the aid of a stethoscope. It is necessary to compress the femoral artery distal to the stethoscope head to produce the characteristic double tone sound.

○ *Hill's sign*
   This is a non-specific sign of aortic regurgitation — it is also seen in other causes of a hyperdynamic circulation, such as thyrotoxicosis, beri-beri, or pregnancy. Check the blood pressures in the upper and lower limbs. If the pressure in the lower limbs exceeds that in the upper limbs by more than 20 mmHg, then the sign is positive.

○ *Quincke's sign*
   Pulsatile blanching of the nail bed.

○ *De Musset's sign*
   Named after the famous French poet whose head nodded in time with his arterial pulsations due to his syphilis related aortic regurgitation.

• **Pulsus paradoxus**
   This is a misnomer. This is an exaggerated physiological phenomenon, rather than a paradox as the name implies. The volume of the pulse rises with expiration, with the increase in stroke volume, and falls during inspiration. When it is present, it suggests either restricted left ventricular filling during inspiration (associated

with a mild increase in pericardial pressure and increased right heart filling that shifts the interventricular septum towards the left ventricle to impair left sided filling) such as in pericardial tamponade, or exaggerated changes in intrathoracic pressure as in severe asthma. Other causes of pulsus paradoxus include right ventricular infarction, large pulmonary embolus, and tense ascites or obesity.

Pulsus paradox is quantified by measuring a change in systolic blood pressure from inspiration to expiration of greater than 12 mmHg or 10% of systolic pressure. To successfully measure this, inflate the brachial cuff pressure to beyond systolic pressure. Palpate the brachial pulse and note the pressure it returns on expiration. Slowly decrease the pulse until you can identify the brachial pulse on inspiration. The difference in systolic pressure is used to estimate the magnitude of pulsus paradox.

- **Pulsus alternans**
  This abnormality describes a pulse that alternates between a larger and smaller volume on a beat to beat basis. This is a regular pulse and is seen in severe cardiac failure.

- **Pulsus bigeminus**
  This is often confused with pulsus alternans. For every other normal beat at a shorter than usual interval there is a lower volume beat, usually due to a premature ventricular contraction. It does not imply severe cardiac failure. A common cause now is Digoxin toxicity.

- **Jerky pulse**
  This is often seen in hypertrophic cardiomyopathy as the hypertrophied ventricle rapidly empties and then quickly drops its output as the outflow pathway is obstructed.

Blood Pressure Assessment

The brachial blood pressure is often performed by others but needs confirmation by the physician at least on the initial visit. Failure to measure or ask for the blood pressure by the student who is being tested for exam technique is a fatal error! Measuring the brachial blood pressure requires attention to technique as outlined below.

A small cuff in relation to the arm size will artificially increase blood pressure readings. A rough rule of thumb is that the width of the cuff should be about half the circumference of the arm. The standard cuff size for a normal adult will be accurate for arm circumferences of up to 27 cm, but larger cuffs will be required for obese patients.

Blood pressure should usually be taken in both arms. A difference of 20 mmHg in systolic pressure between both arms raises the suspicion of subclavian stenosis, an important cause of angina in patients who have had the left internal mammary artery used in coronary artery bypass.

What about aortic dissection? If the patient presents with chest pain and has difference in BP between both arms, think of aortic dissection.

Ideally the blood pressure should be measured in a seated patient after 5–10 minutes of rest, where the cuff is at the level of the heart. If the position is below the heart the pressure will be relatively higher. The converse is also true. Normally the blood pressure remains the same or even increases from the lying to the sitting position, although mean arterial pressure remains the same.

In patients with postural hypotension, the blood pressure will drop on standing by greater than 20 mmHg systolic, and in the elderly may lead to falls and syncope. When testing for postural hypotension, the BP should be taken immediately upon standing and after three minutes of upright position. Take care; patients often collapse during this, watch the patient as well as the sphygmomanometer, and prepare to let the patient lie down immediately if they are going to faint!

Common causes of postural hypotension include hypovolaemia (due to diuretics, dehydration or bleeding), autonomic dysfunction that may be idiopathic or associated with a

> **Kichu's thoughts . . .**
>
> Remember to palpate systolic blood pressure before auscultating — that way you won't miss an auscultatory gap.

systemic illness such as diabetes or Parkinson's disease, or drugs such as L-dopa or vasodilators. Postural hypotension due to hypovolaemia should be associated with a postural tachycardia. Where autonomic dysfunction is the cause, this tachycardic response may not be seen.

Technique of Brachial Blood Pressure Measurement

Place the cuff around the forearm several centimetres above the antecubital fossa. Palpate the radial pulse on the same side and then inflate the cuff until the radial pulse can no longer be detected. Then slowly deflate the cuff and note at what point the pulse becomes detectable again. This is the systolic blood pressure as determined "by palpation" or "palp". Checking the systolic pressure by this means has two advantages. The first is that it is more sensitive in patients with very low blood pressures. The second is that it avoids the problem of the auscultatory gap (see below).

The method for auscultation of the blood pressure was first described by a young surgeon in the Czar's army, Korotkoff. The five sounds heard during auscultation to determine blood pressure are named in his honour. Fully deflate the cuff. Place the diaphragm of the stethoscope over the brachial pulse, which can be located just medial to the biceps tendon in the antecubital fossa. Inflate the cuff till the pressure is above that of systolic pressure determined by palpation. Slowly deflate the cuff. At about the systolic pressure, the artery will allow a small jet of blood through that will be detected by auscultation as a thud. This is referred to as the "Korotkoff I sound". The various sounds heard during further deflation of the cuff are also given the designation Korotkoff with numbers II through V. They are described below. However, they are of fairly limited usefulness except for Korotkoff V, which is where the sound heard over the brachial artery disappears, and occurs at just below the arterial diastolic pressure. Korotkoff IV, where the sound becomes muffled, is a more accurate approximation of diastolic pressure in severe aortic regurgitation. However, Korotkoff V is far more reproducible and is used to indicate diastolic pressure.

The Korotkoff Sounds

These actually correspond to blood pressures:

I — Pressure at which a sound is first heard during the release of the blood pressure cuff.

II — Increase in sound intensity as further pressure is released, sound has a blowing quality.

III — A soft thud as sound decreases in intensity.

IV — Sound becomes muffled.

V — Sound disappears.

Variation in Blood Pressure

Blood pressure varies with activity, anxiety, and pain throughout the day, so it is worthwhile repeating the blood pressure measurement at the end of the examination if it was high at the beginning. As a result, borderline elevations of blood pressure are often confirmed at a later examination before considering antihypertensive therapy.

The blood pressure in patients with atrial fibrillation varies due to the variability in left ventricular filling and ejection. A simple method is to take the Korotkoff I as the pressure where the majority of beats can be heard, and the Korotkoff V as the pressure where the majority of beats have disappeared. Automatic blood pressure readings tend to fluctuate widely from reading to reading, and are probably best abandoned in favour of manual estimation of blood pressure.

Office BP is usually higher than home readings. This is one of the reasons for doing 24-hour ambulatory monitoring.

If you have a patient with difficulty to control BP on medications, first find out whether the patient is taking medication, before initiating investigations. Some patients come to see the doctor without taking the medications on the day of appointment to see whether the BP is under control!

The Auscultatory Gap

This refers to the loss of Korotkoff sounds during deflation of the cuff from the true systolic reading but at pressures higher than that of the true diastolic pressure. The sounds then re-emerge as the cuff is slowly released, only to disappear as pressure falls below the diastolic. The auscultatory gap can lead to marked underestimation of the true systolic pressure. This can be avoided by checking the systolic pressure by palpation before proceeding to the auscultatory method.

Pseudohypertension

This is the phenomenon of falsely elevated blood pressure due to calcified stiff arteries that resist the external pressure of the inflated cuff. Osler described a technique that allows one to test for this condition. First, palpate the radial pulse. Then occlude the artery above this pulse by inflating the cuff of the sphygmomanometer at the antecubital fossa. The pulse will normally no longer be palpable. If the vessel wall is sufficiently stiff though, the artery can be rolled under the finger. A falsely elevated blood pressure reading may well be obtained from such patients (Osler's phenomenon).

Jugular Venous Pressure

The jugular venous pressure (JVP) can yield valuable information about cardiac function (especially of the right ventricle) and pulmonary function, and is an important component of the assessment of volume status. The JVP is most commonly elevated with a raised venous pressure due to cardiac failure or hypervolaemia.

In principle, the JVP reflects the height of the column of venous blood that rises above the physiologic zero point, which corresponds to the right atrium in humans. In practice it is necessary to estimate the position of the right atrium, by one of two techniques:

- **The angle of louis/sternal angle**
  This is the quickest and most commonly used method. The sternal angle lies about 5 cm above the center of the right atrium. In normal persons, the venous column of blood will normally not rise

more than 1 to 2 cm above the sternal angle, irrespective of position (corresponding to a right atrial pressure of about 7 cm H_2O). Therefore, a venous column rising three or more centimetres above the sternal angle is suggestive of a raised right atrial filling pressure.

- **The phlebostatic axis**
  This is the point at the level of the fourth intercostal space midway between anterior and posterior surfaces of the chest. While there is some theoretical advantages to using this point in the estimation of JVP, it is of less value at the bedside simply because it is easier to get agreement between examiners as to the location of the sternal angle.

  An approach to examining the JVP is described below.

A Strategy for Examination of the JVP

The patient is positioned so that the upper body rests at about 45° above horizontal. Good lighting is important, and light falling tangentially on the right neck (e.g. from a torch or flashlight) can help identifiy the JVP. The head is turned slightly towards the left shoulder. Inspect the right side of the neck for the appearance of a double venous flicker just medial to the sternocleidomastoid muscle. The collapse or descent in the venous wave form is often more easily appreciated (whereas an outward pulse is often the carotid pulse). The external jugular is often seen as a cord, and can provide an indication of an elevated JVP, but often does not translate the venous waveform well

Kichu's thoughts . . .

If you start the examination by looking for ankle oedema, you will have an important hint for examining the JVP. If there is ankle oedema, the JVP is more likely to be elevated. If there is no ankle oedema, the JVP is less likely to be raised. There are some exceptions to each of these rules: there may be oedema with a normal JVP in low albumin states and venous obstructions. Oedema may be lacking if the feet have been elevated a few days — even if there is gross right ventricular failure.

due to compression of this vein by external structures. The JVP is easier to see in slim or young people and is is more difficult to see in an obese person, or a person with a short or bull neck.

A markedly high JVP may be missed because the venous flicker is occurring above the angle of the jaw. In this case, the top of the waveform may be seen by sitting the patient up at 90°. Alternatively, look at the patient's earlobes — if these move with the characteristic double flicker of a raised JVP, then the venous column is very likely to be elevated above the angle of the jaw.

- **The abdominojugular reflex**
  If the jugular venous movements are not apparent, apply gentle pressure over the mid-abdomen and look for the JVP at the neck for about 10 seconds. Normally this manoeuvre does not affect the JVP, or if it does so, only for a few seconds. If the JVP rises by 4 or more centimetres and remains elevated for the duration of the abdominal compression, then this is suggestive of raised right atrial pressure or reduced atrial compliance.
- **Kussmaul's sign**
  This is a rise in the JVP seen with inspiration. It is the opposite of what is seen in normal people and this reflects the inability of the heart to compensate for a modest increase in venous return. This sign is classically seen in constrictive pericarditis in association with a raised JVP. This condition was originally described in tuberculous pericarditis and is rarely seen. Kussmaul's sign is also seen in right ventricular infarction, right heart failure, tricuspid stenosis, and restrictive cardiomyopathy. It is not seen in acute cardiac tamponade, although it may be seen if tamponade occurs with a degree of constrictive pericardiditis. Common cause for a Kussmaul's sign nowadays is right ventricular infarction.

Interpretation of the Venous Waveform

The bedside observer can detect two distinct positive waves ("a" and "v") and negative waves, or descents of movement ("x'" and "y"). A third, "c" wave, is seen in venous waveforms measured using transducers ("c" for the positive wave and "x" for the preceding descent).

The "a" wave is produced by contraction of the right atria and is the most prominent. The

> **Kichu's thoughts . . .**
>
> "a" = for atrial contraction
> "c" = for closure of tricuspid
> "v" = for vesticular contractions

following "x" descent occurs during atrial relaxation. After the ventricle begins to contract, initially producing the "c" wave, the prominent "x'" descent is produced as the right atrium is pulled inferiorly by the contracting ventricle. The "v" wave is produced by filling of the right atrium during ventricular systole against a closed tricuspid valve. This is followed by a second prominent "y" descent which is produced during the emptying of the atrium into the ventricle during diastole. Hence the "x'" descent occurs in systole and the "y" descent occurs in diastole. The a wave occurs in late diastole and the "v" wave occurs in late systole.

The individual components of the venous wave may be helped by simultaneously auscultating the heart sounds, or by palpating the carotid pulse to determine systole and diastole. The "x" descent ends just before the S2 (the second heart sound), while the "y" descent begins just after it. The "x'" is systolic and coincides with the carotid pulse, while the "y" is diastolic and begins a short while after the carotid pulse. Now look for the outward waves of movement. Some abnormalities are described below.

Abnormalities of Jugular Venous Waveform

Examples of abnormalities of the descents:

- **"X" < "Y"**
  This is seen in atrial fibrillation, where the "a" wave is lost. Mild tricuspid regurgitation will also result in reduced prominence of the "x'" descent. During ventricular contraction, backflow of ventricular pressure due to an incompetent valve offsets the drop in venous pressure usually produced by downward movement of the atrium.

- **"X'" = "Y"**
  The "x'" descent is usually more prominent than the "y" descent. If they are of approximately equal size, it suggests that the "y" descent is unusually prominent. This is seen in constrictive pericarditis and atrialseptal defect.
- **"Y" absent**
  This may be a normal finding if the JVP is not elevated. Tricuspid stenosis can also result in the disappearance of the "y" descent.
- **Rapid "Y" descent**
  This is a prominent "y" descent in the presence of a normal "x'" descent. It is a good sign of constrictive pericarditis or restrictive disease of the right heart.
- **Abnormalities of the "A" or "V" waves**
  - **Giant "s" waves**
    These precede the S1, and occur with every beat and indicate outflow obstruction such as tricuspid or pulmonary valve stenosis and pulmonary hypertension.
  - **Canon "a" waves**
    These are distinct from giant "a" waves. These occur with dissociation of atrial contraction and ventricular contraction, so that the atria contract against a closed tricuspid valve. Unlike giant "a" waves, canon "a" waves occur only occasionally rather than with every beat.
  - **Tricuspid regurgitation**
    Tricuspid regurgitation, often seen in pulmonary hypertension, is associated with very prominent jugular venous pulsations that lack an "x" or "x'" descent. They consist of a single outward systolic movement that occurs concurrently with the carotid pulse and collapses in early diastole, just after the S2. The absence of an "x" descent allows them to be distinguished from giant "a" waves.

Inspecting the Chest

The apex beat is the lower and lateral most point of the cardiac impulse palpable on the chest wall. It is usually localized with reference to the rib level at which it occurs and with its relationship with the midclavicular line. The midclavicular line is drawn from a point midway along the clavicle and descend vertically downwards, and often does not coincide with the location of the nipple. The apex is usually located in the fifth intercostal space in the midclavicular line. Laterally displacement may be best described with reference to the anterior axillary line or even the midaxillary lines.

- **Patient positioning**
  The apex beat is usually observed with the patient lying at 45° to the horizontal. If not identified, it can sometimes be accentuated by sitting the patient forward or rotating the patient to the left side.
- **Inspection**
  The apex beat can often be seen especially in slim persons. The normal pulse is about 3 cm in diameter. Examine the left and right sides of the chest in case of dextrocardia.
- **Palpation**
  Palpation with the palm of the hand and fingers should start at a lateral position and move more anteriorly in order to avoid missing a displaced beat. A displaced apex beat usually indicates dilation of the left ventricle. Hypertrophy generally does not lead to a displaced apex beat.

Apex Beat

A normal apex beat is about 3–4 cm in diameter, or a little more than 1.5 fingertips. A wider diameter apex beat suggests dilation of the left ventricle.

- **Hyperkinetic apex**
  This is also referred to as hyperdynamic or pressure-loaded apex, a forceful and sustained apical impulse often seen in left ventricular hypertrophy.
- **Sustained apical movement**
  A sustained apex beat suggests cardiomyopathy or severe aortic stenosis.

- **Double apical impulse**

  This is a distinct double movement of the apex with sinus rhythm that may be found in hypertrophic cardiomyopathy, a left ventricular aneurysm involving the anterior wall or apex.

Further Palpation of the Chest Wall

Palpation of the chest wall during a cardiac exam should not end with the palpation of the apex. There is more to be found.

- **Palpating for a left parasternal heave**

  Normally only a slight inward movement is palpable. A sustained outward movement is referred to as a heave. The presence of a left parasternal heave suggests dilation of the right ventricle, an anterior mediastinal structure. It can also be due to marked left atrial dilatation as may be seen in mitral stenosis.

  A systolic downward movement of the right ventricle may also be felt in the epigastrium. This may be palpated by placing the palmar aspect of your thumb under the left costal margin with the tip of the thumb towards the xiphoid process. An enlarged right ventricle can be felt tapping downwards on the surface of the thumb. Sometimes it is necessary to ask the patient to take a deep breath and hold it to palpate the enlarged ventricle.

- **Hyperkinetic movement of the left sternal edge**

  Unlike a left parasternal heave, this is a non-sustained outward movement of the left sternal edge. This is most commonly due to a hyperdynamic circulation, for example due to fever, but it may be a sign of an atrial septal defect — in this circumstance then it is caused by increased filling of the right ventricle. Look for the fixed splitting of the second heart sound, a prominent "y" descent in the neck veins, a soft systolic murmur in the second left intercostal space, as other signs to support this diagnosis.

- **Hyperkinetic movement of the right parasternal edge**

  This is found in severe tricuspid regurgitation or mitral regurgitation. In the former it is due to expansion of the right atrium and liver, in the latter dilation of the left atrium is the cause.

- **Left parasternal movement in severe mitral regurgitation**
  In patients with very severe mitral regurgitation, the left atrium of the heart can become massively dilated, and its rapid filling during ventricular contraction can push the heart forward, creating a late systolic left parasternal impulse. This occurs even when the right ventricle, which overlies the left atrium, is of normal dimensions.
- **Thrills**
  A thrill is a vibration-like movement of the chest wall caused by turbulent blood flow over a heart valve. It is a palpable murmur. Thrills are usually best palpated using the distal palm. Aortic and pulmonary stenotic lesions produce murmurs that are best felt with the patient leaning forward and in full expiration.
- **A palpable P2**
  A palpable pulmonary component of the second heart sound (P2) is considered a sign of pulmonary hypertension. It is felt with the fingertips as a tapping movement. Palpate over the pulmonary area of the chest — the left sternal edge, second intercostal space, again with the patient sitting forward.

Percussion in the Cardiac Examination

This has generally fallen from favour as part of the routine cardiac examination, because it adds little to the exam.

Auscultation of the Heart

This is one of the most challenging and rewarding components of the physical examination.

- **The stethoscope**
  The stethoscope should have both a bell — a shallow metal cup used to auscultate low frequency sounds, and a diaphragm — a bell covered by a metal or plastic sheet which is used especially for higher frequency sounds. The ear buds need to fit snugly as air leak allows in background noise from the room and substantially impairs performance of the stethoscope.

Kichu's thoughts . . .

By the time you are about to start to auscultate you may already have
a good idea about what you are likely to hear. It is much easier to
listen for something rather than just listening in the hope you may hear
something. After you have felt for the left ventricle (the apex beat) and
the right ventricle (a left sternal heave), you should be able to have a
fairly good idea of whether either ventricle is enlarged. Many of the
common valvular abnormalities lead to enlarged ventricles, and you
will have a much better idea of what could be wrong:

	Common conditions	Less common conditions
Big left ventricle	Mitral regurgitation Aortic regurgitation (Not common in aortic stenosis except in end stage)	End-stage ischaemic heart disease (IHD) End-stage hypertension End-stage aortic stenosis
Big right ventricle	Tricuspid regurgitation Pulmonary hypertensions from • Mitral stenosis • Lung disease	Most congenital heart diseases Pulmonary stenosis
Both ventricles big	Combined valvular disease Congestive cardiac failure	Dilated cardiomyopathy from • Alcohol • Viral • Hereditary • Idiopathic
Neither ventricle big	Mitral stenosis Aortic stenosis	

- **Positioning the patient**

  The patient is best examined in a quiet environment. The patient
  may need to be moved through several positions in the course of
  a typical auscultation of the cardiovascular system. Initially the
  patient should be lying at 45° to the horizontal. Clothing should
  be removed, but a sheet or gown may be placed over the breasts
  of female patients for modesty before and after inspecting the

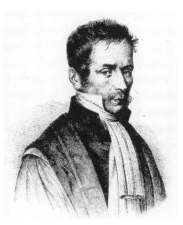

Historical Aside: The Origin of the Stethoscope

The stethoscope was first developed in France in 1816 by René-Théophile-Hyacinthe Laennec, who used a rolled-up "quire of paper" in order to auscultate the heart of a young woman. Prior to this, doctors auscultated the heart by placing the ear directly to the chest wall.

Later, Laennec used a stethoscope that consisted of a wooden tube and was monaural. His device was similar to the ear trumpet, a historical form of hearing aid. Indeed, his invention was almost indistinguishable in structure and function from the trumpet, then known as a "microphone". In 1851, Arthur Leared invented a binaural stethoscope, and in 1852 George Cammann perfected the design of the instrument for commercial production, which has become the standard ever since. Cammann also authored a major treatise on diagnosis by auscultation, which the refined binaural stethoscope made possible. Numerous designs now exist, including electronic models. A standard acoustic model performs well in the hands and ears of a skilled clinician and most designs have their adherents.

precordium. The examiner should take time to explain to the patient what they are doing as anxiety may increase the heart rate, complicating auscultation. The patient should be told to keep quiet too, since some patients want to continue the history while you are auscultating!

An Approach to Auscultation

A systematic approach is very important, but the approach used will vary between examiners. Some choose to examine the typical areas from the top down and others vice versa. Our approach is described here.

Begin with the bell of the stethoscope over the apex. The stethoscope should be applied gently, as too forceful a pressure will cause the skin to stretch over the bell and create a dia-

Kichu's thoughts . . .

Don't forget that the most important part of the stethoscope is what lies between the ear pieces.

phragm. The first and second heart sounds are usually low frequency sounds, best heard with the bell. The first heart sound coincides with the closure of the mitral and tricuspid valves, and is probably due to vibrations in the heart and within the column of blood rather than the closure of the valves themselves. The first sound may be split, but is usually audible as a single sound. It occurs at the beginning of systole — the beginning of the carotid pulse. The second heart sound is caused by the closure of the aortic and pulmonary valves. It is often split, due to the lower pressures in the pulmonary circulation resulting in a slight relative delay in pulmonary valve closure with respect to the aortic valve. The second sound occurs at the beginning of diastole. The first and second sounds are sometimes imitated using the onomatopoeia of "lub dup", "lub dup", "lub dup" where S1 is "lub" and S2 is "dup". These heart sounds are discussed in more detail in later sections. Listen for the presence of third or fourth heart sounds. The third heart sound tends to be a low frequency sound.

The sounds of mitral stenosis are best heard at the apex with a bell. As they can be very soft, an opening snap may require the patient to be rolled into the left lateral decubitus position to hear the diastolic murmur of mitral stenosis.

Now engage the diaphragm of the stethoscope and listen at the apex again. Move the diaphragm to the lower left sternal edge (tricuspid region), left sternal edge (left ventricular outflow tract), upper left sternal edge (pulmonary area) and upper right sternal edge (aortic area). Concentrate on the heart sounds and any deviations from

Kichu's thoughts . . .

Remember that the patient has to breathe (and often short of breath), so don't ask them to stop breathing for too long. A good practice is to hold your breath at the same time as the patient.

normal, for example, listen for splitting of the second heart sound in the pulmonary area which changes with respiration. This splitting is accentuated by inspiration, as increased right heart filling delays closure of the pulmonary valve further.

In each region, focus on systole and diastole separately and note the quality as well as loudness of extra sounds and murmurs. Aortic regurgitation and left ventricular outflow tract murmurs are often best heard using the diaphragm of the stethoscope with the patient sitting up and leaning forward in expiration.

A murmur identified at the upper sternum should be followed into the subclavian region and neck to note the radiation of a murmur. Recall that bruits from obstructive disease of the great vessels may also be confused with cardiac murmurs.

The First Heart Sound

The S1 is usually louder in conditions where systole starts with the mitral and tricuspid valves widely open. For example, after exercise or in hyperdynamic states (thyrotoxicosis or fever), tachycardia leads to reduced ventricular filling time and widely open valves at the onset of systole that close forcefully with ventricular contraction. A loud S1 is also produced with mitral and tricuspid stenosis because ventricular filling is delayed. A loud S1 should alert the examiner to the possibility of mitral stenosis and prompt positional changes to accentuate the diastolic murmur. A soft S1 may occur with prolonged diastolic filling or mitral or tricuspid regurgitation where the valves do not oppose correctly in systole. Acute and severe aortic regurgitation may result in a soft S1 due to a rapid rise in left ventricular end-diastolic pressure that starts to close the mitral valve before systole.

The Second Heart Sound

The pulmonary component of the second heart sound (P2) is louder in pulmonary hypertension and the aortic component (A2) of the second heart sound is louder with systemic hypertension.

The second heart sound may be split normally with P2 being delayed compared to A2 due to the lower pulmonary artery pressure compared to systemic pressure. Splitting with delay of the P2 is normally accentuated by inspiration, or any cause of increased right ventricular pressures (e.g. ventricular septal defect (VSD) and pulmonary stenosis) or right bundle branch block (delayed activation of the right ventricle): fixed splitting without respiratory variation occurs with an atrial septal defect, and reverse splitting (narrowing of the split with inspiration and widening in expiration) occurs with elevated left ventricular pressures (aortic stenosis) or left bundle branch block.

The Third Heart Sound

It is a low-pitched noise heard in early to mid-diastole which follows closely after the S2. It has a cadence that has the similar "y" in Kentuck-y (with "Ken" being S1 and "tuck" S2). The left ventricular S3 is best heard with the patient in the left lateral decubitus position with the bell gently applied. The S3 and S4 are often called a "gallop rhythm" due to their sound resembling a horse gallop.

The third heart sound is thought to be due to rapid diastolic filling or reduced left ventricular compliance. It is often normal in children and young adults, but considered pathological in older adults.

The Fourth Heart Sound

This is also referred to as the S4. This is a higher-pitched sound than S3, best heard with the lightly applied bell of the stethoscope at the apex or left lower sternum. It can originate from either the left or the right ventricle of the heart and occurs before S1. The cadence of S4 is similar to "Tenn" in Tenn-e-see (with "e" being S1 and "see" being S2).

The S4 is also called the atrial gallop, although the sound is produced in a poorly compliant ventricle because of forceful atrial filling. As a result, it is never heard in atrial fibrillation, nor can the left heart produce it if there is mitral stenosis.

The S4 is due to reduced ventricular compliance, and therefore ventricular hypertrophy is a common cause. In the presence of angina or acute myocardial infarction, the ventricle also becomes stiff, potentially inducing an S4. An S4 may also be heard after completed myocardial infarction due to increased fibrosis of the vessel wall. The sound is not heard in constrictive pericarditis or cardiac tamponade due to decreased movement of the ventricle.

In tachycardia, an S3 and S4 may run together, causing a summation gallop.

Other Heart Sounds

- **The opening snap**
  This is heard in mitral or tricuspid stenosis, and is a loud, high-pitched sound frequently heard in early diastole. It is generated as the stenosed mitral valve leaflets open fully and then suddenly stop. It is then followed by the soft, low-pitched rumbling diastolic murmur of mitral or tricuspid stenosis. The opening snap tends to occur later in diastole than the P2 component of the second heart sound and is a higher frequency than S3. The opening snap occurs earlier in diastole with more severe mitral stenosis.
- **The pericardial knock**
  This has some similarities to the third heart sound in that it is caused by a sudden cessation of expansion of the ventricle during diastole — some authors refer to it as a variant form of the S3. It is caused by constrictive pericarditis, where the pericardial sac is diseased and limits ventricular movement. It is a high-pitched, loud, early diastolic sound often heard at the apex and left sternal edge. It is later in diastole than the opening snap or the A2, and is earlier than the S3.
- **The tumour plop**
  The tumour plop is heard in the presence of an atrial myxoma that is prolapsing into the left ventricle during diastole. The sound varies in its timing, and may be identified between early and mid-diastole.

- **Prosthetic heart sounds**

  These sounds are common and reflect the type of prosthetic valve present, its position, and pathological states. Ball valves will produce distinct, metallic, opening and closing clicks, while disk valves tend to produce a closing click. Short systolic murmurs are usually associated with prosthetic valves in the aortic position. However, continuous murmurs or diastolic murmurs are often pathological.

Murmurs

Murmurs are described according to their timing in the cardiac cycle, location where they are loudest, pattern or shape, intensity, radiation and response to dynamic manoeuvres.

- **Timing**

  The first and second heart sounds are the reference for timing of the murmur. The location in diastole and systole (early, middle, late) are used to describe the location of the murmurs in the phase of the cardiac cycle.

  Continuous murmurs occur with communication between two regions with a continuous pressure gradient (e.g. patent ductus arteriosus).

- **Pattern or shape**

  This refers to a graphical representation of the intensity of the murmur over time of the murmur. The two most common shapes for systolic murmurs are the crescendo–decrescendo (diamond-shaped) murmur and the pansystolic murmur. Ejection murmurs from the aortic or pulmonic valves tend to be crescendo–decrescendo in pattern, whereas systolic murmurs from the tricuspid or mitral valves are more continuous in pattern, although their timing may only occur in part of systole.

  Most diastolic murmurs have a decrescendo pattern.

- **Radiation**

  Auscultate over the axilla and over the carotid arteries, which are common sites of radiation of the murmurs of mitral insufficiency and aortic stenosis, respectively.

- Pitch
  This is the tone of the murmur, which can be either high or low pitched, usually reflecting the pressure gradient and the size of the valve aperture through which the murmur is generated.
- Timbre
  This refers to whether the murmur is harsh or has a musical quality. Various colourful descriptions of the timbre of a murmur can be found in the literature.
- Intensity
  The intensity of a murmur can be graded from 1 to 6, using the Levine grading system. This is essentially a measure of how loud a murmur is.

Grade 1: The murmur is barely audible — it is not heard if auscultated only for a moment.

Grade 2: The murmur is faint, but can be heard as soon as the stethoscope is applied to the chest wall.

Grade 3: A murmur that is louder than Grade 2, but is not associated with a thrill.

Grade 4: The murmur is readily audible — it is associated with a faint thrill.

Grade 5: The murmur is loud, and associated with a readily palpable thrill.

Grade 6: The murmur is very loud and can be heard with the stethoscope held a few centimetres from the chest.

> **Kichu's thoughts . . .**
>
> Grading of the murmur depends on the grading of the physician.

Dynamic Manoeuvres

Several dynamic manoeuvres are used to distinguish various murmurs. Slow, exaggerated breathing can distinguish murmurs from right sided chambers that increase with right sided filling, whereas expiration tends to accentuate murmurs from left sided chambers. Expiration and leaning the patient forward will also accentuate aortic incompetence as the distance between the heart and the sternum is decreased.

The Valsalva manoeuvre in the midphase increases intrathoracic pressure, reduces cardiac filling and tends to soften most murmurs. However, the systolic murmur of hypertrophic obstructive cardiomyopathy is increased because the left ventricular volume is lower and this accentuates the outflow obstruction. At this time the click of mitral valve prolapse moves earlier.

Squatting increases arterial resistance, venous return, as well as stroke volume and chamber size. This tends to accentuate murmurs. However, the increased left ventricular volume decreases the murmur of hypertrophic cardiomyopathy and delays the click of mitral valve prolapse. Isometric exercise (e.g. fist clench) has a similar but less pronounced effect.

Characteristics of Murmurs

- **Mitral regurgitation**
  The murmur of mitral regurgitation (MR) is one of the most common cardiac murmurs identified at the bedside. It is usually a pansystolic murmur which is loudest at the apex of the heart. It can radiate to the axilla and sometimes to the left subscapular area. Rarely, an isolated incompetence of the medial portion of the posterior leaflet, the murmur can radiate to the aortic area and even to the carotids, mimicking the murmur of aortic stenosis.

Coexisting findings can help in this diagnosis. In mitral regurgitant murmurs, look for:

- ○ A normal S1. Contrary to common belief, a soft S1 is found in about 10% of patients with mitral regurgitation, 10% have a loud S1, and in the majority the S1 is normal.
- ○ A left ventricular S3 — found in about 90% of those with severe MR.
- ○ A displaced and enlarged apex beat.
- ○ A left parasternal movement from an enlarged left atrium.
- ○ A hyperkinetic arterial pulse.

The most useful signs of severe mitral regurgitation are:

1. The intensity of the murmur — usually Grade 3 or greater (positive likelihood ratio 4.4).
2. The presence of an S3 (positive likelihood ratio 1.8). The louder the S3, the greater the severity of the valvular lesion.
3. The presence of a left parasternal impulse in the absence of signs of right ventricular strain or mitral stenosis (see below for the signs of this valvular lesion).
4. A more widely displaced apex, suggesting more severe MR.
5. Widely split S2. In the absence of severe pulmonary hypertension, the more widely split the S2, the worse the mitral regurgitation S2.

The murmur of aortic stenosis can sometimes mimic that of mitral regurgitation. Aortic stenosis typically produces a harsh, rough sounding murmur which changes across the chest towards the apex of the heart so that it sounds more like the high pitched musical sound of mitral regurgitation. This is referred to as the Gallavardin phenomenon.

- **Aortic stenosis**
  The murmur of aortic stenosis is usually a rough, harsh sounding murmur, rather like the sound of a person clearing his throat. It is usually loudest at the right second intercostal space. It often radiates to the neck and may be heard over the carotid arteries.

  Features on history that suggest severe aortic stenosis include syncope, exertional dyspnoea and exertional angina. An ECG demonstrating left ventricular hypertrophy is also supportive.

  Useful signs of severe aortic stenosis, including the positive likelihood ratios (LR), are given below:

1. An absent A2 (LR 4.5)
2. Late peaking murmur (LR 4.4)
3. Sustained apical impulse (LR 4.1)
4. Prolonged murmur (LR 3.9)
5. Pulsus tardus: Delayed carotid artery upstroke (LR 3.7)

6. Apical carotid delay: Palpable delay between the apical and carotid impulse (LR 2.6)
7. Brachioradial delay: Palpable delay between the brachial and radial arterial pulses (LR 2.5)
8. Radiation of the murmur to the neck (LR 1.4)

The loudness of the murmur, the presence of an S3 or S4 and the reverse splitting of the second sound or the presence of an ejection click are not helpful signs in distinguishing severity.

The development of cardiac failure with a reduced stroke volume may lead to a reduction in the intensity of the murmur of even severe aortic stenosis.

- **Mitral stenosis**
  The murmur of mitral stenosis is often quite difficult to hear — but very important nonetheless and not to be missed. It is a soft murmur, with a low pitched rumbling sound that is best heard with the bell of the stethoscope and the patient rolled into the left lateral position over the apex. It is best heard in expiration. It

---

CASE STUDY 3.3

A 53-year-old business woman with no significant past medical problems presents with breathlessness when walking up steps.

She is a non-smoker and takes hormone replacement therapy for menopausal symptoms.

She appears well. Her pulse is 80 beats per minute and has a small volume. There is a delayed carotid upstroke. The blood pressure is 110/70. Her apex beat is vigorous and slightly displaced. She has a harsh, low pitched murmur at the left sternal edge and aortic area with radiation to the carotids. There is an S4 with a noticeably soft A2.

Her chest is clear and there is no sacral or pedal oedema.

What diagnosis or diagnoses do these signs and history suggest?
How serious is the problem?
What would a click preceding the murmur imply?

begins just after the opening snap, and therefore shortly after the second heart sound. You should suspect this valvular lesion, and therefore roll the patient onto the left side for every patient in whom you hear a loud S1.

The diagnosis is as always, assisted by the company the murmur keeps. The following signs are often associated with the murmur of mitral stenosis:

1. A reduced pulse pressure and blood pressure.
2. Atrial fibrillation.
3. JVP may be normal. There may be a prominent "a" wave if it is pulmonary hypertension.
4. A tapping apex beat may be present — this is essentially a palpable S1.
5. A diastolic thrill may very rarely be palpated with the patient rolled onto the left lateral position.

If mitral stenosis is severe, look for the following signs:

1. A small or low volume pulse.
2. A soft first heart sound due to immobile valve cusps.
3. Long diastolic murmur.
4. A diastolic thrill at the apex.
5. Signs of pulmonary hypertension.

- **Tricuspid regurgitation**
  This is an important and not uncommon heart valve defect with a characteristic mumur. The characterisitics of the murmur and the associated features depend on the pressures within the pulmonary system. The most commonly encountered situation is one in which tricuspid regurgitation occurs concurrently with pulmonary hypertension. This results in regurgitation occurring under high pressure. Tricuspid regurgitation due to a valvular lesion in the absence of pulmonary hypertension results in a low pressure regurgitation. The murmur is usually loudest at the lower left sternal edge. As the altered venous return is associated with respiration, the mumur is usually louder on inspiration. This is true of most right sided heart mumurs.

The murmur is usually pansystolic, low pitched and often relatively soft. In some patients, the right ventricle is so enlarged that the left ventrcle is displaced and the murmur in fact becomes loudest at the apex of the heart. It then becomes important to distinguish the mumur from that of mitral regurgitation, which can often be done by considering the associated signs and the specific characteristics of the murmur — the enhancement of the murmur with inspiration, the presence of the murmur at the lower left sternal edge, the presence of an elevated JVP with prominent "v" waves, and a pulsatile liver — all argue for the presence of tricuspid regurgitation over that of isolated mitral regurgitation.

Few signs are associated with tricuspid regurgitation in the presence of low right sided pressures. The neck veins and apex position are typically normal and there are ususally no signs of cardiac failure.

Signs commonly associated with the more common situation of tricuspid regurgitation in the presence of high pulmonary arterial pressures include:

1. A raised JVP with prominent "v" waves.
2. Enhancement of the murmur with inspiration or with application of abdominal pressure.
3. A retracting movement of the apex beat during systole may be detected (in about 20% of patients) in the presence of severe tricuspid regurgitation.
4. A pulsatile liver is a common finding, as are ascites and peripheral oedema.

- **Tricuspid stenosis**
  This is an infrequent valvular lesion and its associated murmur is very rare. The size of the tricuspid valve is large; consequently there are relatively few conditions able to induce sufficient obstruction to the valve to be clinically significant. Rheumatic heart disease is the most common pathology causing tricuspid stenosis.

Fatigue (due principally to decreased cardiac output) and the symptoms of raised systemic venous pressure are dominant. Patients often complain of oedema, or symptoms of hepatic distension and/or ascites.

Typically, one hears a low-pitched diastolic murmur along the left sternal border in the third and fourth intercostal spaces. The murmur is often enhanced by inspiration. In sinus rhythm, it is most prominent at end diastole, whereas in atrial fibrillation, it is usually more prominent in early and mid-diastole. An opening snap can sometimes be heard along the lower left sternal border.

The other physical findings due to tricuspid stenosis are:

1. An abnormally large "a" wave in the jugular venous pulse.
2. The "v" wave, except when tricuspid regurgitation is also present, is normal or reduced, and the "y" descent is slow or absent.
3. If the right atrium is very large, an impulse can be felt in diastole along the lower right sternal border.

The right ventricular lift seen in many patients with tricuspid regurgitation is not present in patients with an isolated tricuspid stenosis. In fact, as most cases of tricuspid stenosis occur in the presence of concurrent mitral stenosis, the signs of mitral stenosis such as the diastolic murmur, the loud first heart sound, and opening snap at the apex may dominate. Look for elevation of the jugular venous pressure in the absence of other signs of pulmonary congestion, as a clue to the presence of tricuspid stenosis in the presence of a mitral stenosis. Also listen for enhancement of the diastolic murmur along the lower left sternal border that will not be detectable in mitral stenosis without the presence of tricuspid stenosis.

One well-documented cause of tricuspid stenosis is the carcinoid syndrome. You should suspect this if you identify tricuspid stenosis in the presence of a large nodular liver. A characteristic facial flush — usually a ruddy, cyanotic appearance may also be noted intermittently.

- **Pulmonary regurgitation**

  Again, this is not a common murmur but an especially important one! The patient may present with symptoms of the condition that has caused pulmonary valve incompetence — the symptoms of an underlying pulmonary disease or of pulmonary hypertension, the carcinoid syndrome or of endocarditis. Isolated pulmonary regurgitation may be asymptomatic even if quite severe, or it may present with breathlessness or fatigue. Some patients develop non-exertional chest pains in the left upper chest, possibly related to the force with which the dilated right ventricle and enlarged pulmonary artery strike the chest wall. A murmur is typically detected as a diastolic murmur along the left sternal border in the second and third interspaces. The murmur may increase in intensity during inspiration and may be very localised. With isolated pulmonary valve regurgitation, this murmur starts following a brief pause after the aortic second sound (in mid-diastole) and is usually short and low pitched. The pulmonary second sound may be audible before the diastolic murmur. If the pulmonary valve cusp is fibrotic and retracted, the pulmonary second sound may be absent. Other findings in isolated pulmonary regurgitation include:

  1. A prominent right ventricular anterior precordial lift.
  2. A lift in the second left interspace which is caused by the dilated pulmonary artery and its exaggerated expansion due to the increased right ventricular stroke volume. Chronic pulmonary hypertension can cause the pulmonary valve to become incompetent. In this situation, the characteristic findings are somewhat different from those of isolated pulmonary regurgitation. The decrescendo murmur occurs in early diastole and is high pitched, loudest in the second interspace and begins immediately after the loud P2. This is called the Graham Steell murmur. Associated features include:

     a. Elevation of the JVP.
     b. If the pulmonary regurgitant volume is large, an early-peaking systolic ejection murmur ending before the second heart sound may be heard. This murmur is quite common,

and is associated with a thrill in 10% of the patients who have it. It can be mistaken for pulmonary stenosis.

c. Abnormal S2 splitting.

d. A right-sided gallop.

Distinguishing pulmonary regurgitation from aortic regurgitation can sometimes be difficult — attenuation of the intensity of the murmur of aortic regurgitation after exposure to the drug amyl nitrate may be useful. This agent does not affect the murmur of pulmonary regurgitation. The absence of peripheral signs of aortic regurgitation should suggest the possibility of pulmonary stenosis in the presence of an appropriate murmur.

- **Pulmonary stenosis**
Most patients with pulmonary stenosis are asymptomatic, but may complain of chest pain or palpitations. There is an ejection systolic murmur that is loudest at the second and third interspaces at the left sternal edge. There is a fairly good correlation between the severity of the murmur and the degree of stenosis, although a very tight stenosis may result in a soft, high-pitched murmur. The greater the degree of severity of the stenosis, the later the murmur peaks. There is radiation to the carotids, but to a lesser extent than what is seen in aortic stenosis. The murmur increases in intensity with inspiration.

Features associated with severe aortic stenosis include:

1. Right ventricular hypertrophy.
2. A precordial lift due to right ventricular hypertrophy.
3. A right-sided fourth heart sound.
4. Jugular venous pressure wave reveals a prominent "a" wave.
5. Widened splitting of the second heart sound due to a later P2. The wideness of the split correlates with the severity of the stenosis.

There may an associated murmur of tricuspid regurgitation.
- **Aortic regurgitation**
This valvular lesion is typically associated with an early diastolic decrescendo murmur. The murmur has a blowing quality and is

of quite a high frequency. There may be a musical quality to the sound, sometimes referred to as a diastolic whoop. The murmur of aortic regurgitation is best heard in the left parasternal area in the third or fourth intercostal space. Often it is difficult to hear. The patient should be positioned forward and asked to breathe out while the examiner auscultates at the lower left sternal edge with the diaphragm of the stethoscope applied firmly to the chest wall. This improves the murmur's audibility. In some patients the murmur is best heard over the cardiac apex or over the mid-precordium. The murmur usually begins at the A2 sound and ends before the S1, although the duration is variable.

The murmur in aortic regurgitation is a particularly useful diagnostic sign. The presence of the characteristic murmur strongly suggests the presence of aortic regurgitation, and the absence of the murmur also argues strongly against the presence of moderate to severe aortic regurgitation.

There are in fact two other murmurs that may be associated with severe aortic regurgitation. These are:

1. A short ejection systolic flow murmur resulting from the very high stroke volume seen in this lesion. It is loudest over the aortic area and left sternal edge. It can be distinguished from the murmur of aortic stenosis by the absence of signs of the latter condition, and the presence of signs of severe aortic incompetence.
2. The Austin Flint murmur — an apical diastolic murmur that can be heard in 60% of patients with severe aortic regurgitation. It resembles the murmur of mitral stenosis, despite the presence of a normal mitral valve. It is loudest just before the S1, unlike the murmur of aortic regurgitation which is loudest just after the S2 and then fades away. The mechanism of the Austin Flint murmur is not known, although various hypotheses have been proposed.

It may be possible to distinguish clinically between the murmurs caused by aortic valvular incompetence and the murmur caused by aortic root dilatation. In aortic root dilatation, the murmur may be loudest at the right sternal edge due to the eccentricity of the regurgitant jet. The same prominence of the murmur over the right chest may be heard in endocarditis where a single cusp of the valve has been destroyed. Prominence of the regurgitant murmur over the right chest has a likelihood ratio of 8.2 for the presence of endocarditis or aortic root dilatation. A number of findings argue for the degree of severity of chronic aortic regurgitation in a patient with the characteristic murmur.

1. The more severe the regurgitation, the louder the murmur — a murmur of Grade 3 or more indicates moderate to severe regurgitation with a likelihood ratio of 8.2.
2. A diastolic blood pressure of less than 50 mmHg in the presence of the characteristic murmur argues for moderate to severe aortic regurgitation with a high likelihood ratio. A diastolic blood pressure of more than 70 mmHg argues against such a lesion.
3. A pulse pressure of greater than 80 mmHg in the presence of the characteristic murmur argues for moderate to severe aortic regurgitation with a high degree of likelihood. A pulse pressure of less than 60 mmHg argues against the diagnosis.
4. Hills test. Quite an easy and useful test to do. It is described above.
5. An enlarged and sustained apex beat is found in nearly all patients with moderate to severe aortic regurgitation — if it is not present, this argues against the diagnosis.

Somewhat confusingly, the situation in acute aortic regurgitation is quite different. In this situation, the left ventricle has not had time to dilate and therefore remains relatively noncompliant. Pressures in the pulmonary system and pulmonary artery are higher. Clinical signs include:

1. A shorter diastolic murmur than in chronic aortic incompetence.

2. Lower pulse pressure — mean about 55 mmHg.
3. Relative tachycardia average 110 beats per minute versus 71 beats per minute in the chronic condition.
4. A soft first heart sound, due to early closure of the mitral valve.
5. A non-displaced apex beat.

- **Atrial septal defect**
  A right-sided ejection systolic murmur may sometimes be detected in atrial septal defect with a large left-to-right shunt. This occurs because of increased flow across the pulmonary valve. Other signs of an atrial septal defect include wide fixed splitting of the S2 and evidence of right ventricular overload. Increased flow across the pulmonary valve associated with increased flow due to hyperthyroidism may also be linked to an ejection systolic murmur.
- **Ventricular septal defect**
  This is a pansystolic murmur heard best over the third and fourth intercostal spaces of the chest wall. It is caused by the flow of blood from the left ventricle to the right across the pressure gradient that exists between the ventricles during systole. The S2 is usually normal and there may be an associated thrill. The intensity of the murmur does not correlate with the size of the ventricular defect — a loud murmur may be generated by high flow velocity over a very small defect which is haemodynamically insignificant.

  The murmur does not alter in intensity with inspiration, which helps to differentiate it from the murmur of tricuspid regurgitation. It does not radiate to the axilla, which helps to distinguish it from the murmur of mitral regurgitation. In the presence of a large left-to-right shunt, there may be a widened split of the S2. There may also be an audible S3 and in some cases, a diastolic murmur relating to increased flow across the mitral valve may also be detected.

  Sometimes, drugs have been used to help distinguish murmurs — since the advent of echocardiography this is almost never done. In the past, distinguishing between the murmurs of a ventricular septal defect and of mitral valve regurgitation has been difficult. Amyl nitrate is not useful for this purpose. Nitroglycerine and sodium nitroprusside can cause a greater reduction of pulmonary vascular resistance than of systemic resistance and, therefore, may cause an increase in the magnitude of left-to-right shunt and the intensity of the murmur in ventricular septal defect.

- **Mammary soufflé**

  A diastolic murmur can sometimes be heard at the left sternal border in pregnant patients. The murmur is usually generated by increased diastolic flow through the internal mammary artery. This sound may be referred to as a "mammary soufflé". This may persist in lactating mothers, even after delivery. Because there can also be a widened pulse pressure in late pregnancy due to decreased peripheral vascular resistance and lower diastolic pressures, some peripheral signs that are associated with aortic regurgitation may occasionally be seen in the company of the "mammary soufflé", including Quincke's sign and pulsatile fingertips.

  Sometimes it is difficult to exclude aortic valvular disease in this situation without resorting to echocardiography.

Pericardial Rub

Although not a murmur, the pericardial rub is an important clinical sign which is often detected during the process of cardiac auscultation. It is a rough sound, originally described as being like the "crackling of new leather". It is usually best heard at the left sternal edge with the diaphragm at the left sternal edge and the patient leaning forward in full expiration. Sometimes the rub may become louder with inspiration. Some rubs can even be palpated.

Unlike most murmurs, rubs may be heard in more than one phase of the cardiac cycle. As many as 85% of cases have both systolic and diastolic components, with the remainder having only a systolic component.

There are many causes of pericardial rubs. These include recent acute myocardial infarction, viral infections, neoplasia, uraemia and connective tissue disorders.

Hypertrophic Cardiomyopathy

This is an important diagnosis to make. The murmur is produced by obstruction to the aortic outflow tract below the level of the valve. The obstruction is between the anterior leaflet of the mitral valve and the hypertrophic interventricular septum. This condition usually generates a harsh midsystolic murmur best heard at the left sternal edge. Unlike most systolic murmurs, the murmur of hypertrophic cardiomyopathy is made louder by manoeuvres that decrease venous return to the heart. Hence when examining a patient with a systolic murmur, one should consider performing the following to look for change in the intensity of the murmur:

1. Valsalva manoeuvre — the finding of a systolic murmur that intensifies with Valsalva has a high positive likelihood ratio for hypertrophic cardiomyopathy.
2. A murmur that becomes louder as one moves from a squatting position to standing has a high positive likelihood ratio for hypertrophic cardiomyopathy. A systolic murmur that becomes softer when moving from a standing to a squatting position is also strongly suggestive of this condition.
3. A systolic murmur that becomes softer with passive leg raising is quite a sensitive and specific finding for hypertrophic cardiomyopathy.
4. Isometric hand grip — if the characteristic murmur becomes softer with this manoeuvre, this suggests hypertrophic cardiomyopathy.

Other findings that can be associated with hypertrophic cardiomyopathy include:

1. A sustained palpable apex beat.

2. A hyperkinetic pulse.
3. A fourth heart sound (found in more than a half of patients with this condition).

Examining the Lung Fields

Before finishing auscultation, the lung fields should be examined to look for signs of cardiac failure (see Chapter 2 on Respiratory Examination).

Examine the Legs and Sacrum

The examination of the lower limbs requires the examiner to ask that the patient's shoes and socks be removed and the limbs exposed. Again, a gown or towel can be draped over the perineum for modesty.

Inspection of the limbs will reveal rashes associated with vasculitis and signs of arterial or venous insufficiency. Arterial insufficiency may be associated with a lack of hair on the limb that also appears to have thin shiny skin and occasionally a coolness to touch. Venous insufficiency is best assessed in the lying and standing positions to note varicosities, as well as the brawny induration associated with inspissated blood cells breaking down in the skin to release hemosiderin. Tendon xanthomata are characteristically present over the Achilles tendon and may be better appreciated by palpation.

Oedema is assessed by gentle but continuous pressure over a bone for several seconds. Pitting oedema is seen in heart failure, although this may become non-pitting with fibrotic changes in the lymphatics over time. In addition, sacral oedema may be apparent, particularly if the patient has been in bed for a long time.

The feet should be inspected for ulcers. Ulcers in patients with diabetes or atherosclerosis affecting the peripheral arteries or due to venous insufficiency constitute an important cause of morbidity.

Arterial Insufficiency

See examination of the "vascular system".

Venous Insufficiency

The patients' legs should be examined while they are in standing and lying positions. While standing the veins over the long and short saphenous distribution are observed and palpated for varicosities. The superficial long saphenous vein runs in the medial aspect of the leg to the groin. The superficial short saphenous vein runs on the posterior margin of the calf from the ankle to the knee.

The superficial veins join the deep veins at the saphenofemoral valve just below the inguinal ligament in the groin, but also through perforating veins along their length. The competence of the saphenofemoral valve can be assessed by the Trendelenburg's test, where the valve is compressed by pressure on the groin with the leg elevated. The patient stands while compression on the groin is applied continuously. If the varicose veins in the leg do not recurr on standing, the valve is incompetent. If the varicosities return during compression of the groin, the perforator veins are incompetent.

A variation of this test uses a ligature around the upper thigh and calf to localise which perforators are incompetent. If the varicosities only return on release of the ligature, the valves of the superficial veins are incompetent.

More detailed description is given in Chapter 8.

Examine the Abdomen

The patient should lie down in the supine position and be examined for signs of right heart failure or other vascular disease. (See Chapter 4 on gastrointestinal examination.)

An enlarged liver or pulsatile liver can indicate right heart failure or severe tricuspid incompetence. In prolonged and severe cases, this may lead to jaundice and chronic liver disease (cardiac jaundice). Splenomegaly may indicate infective endocarditis. The examiner should rest the hand on the abdomen to note any pulsation that could indicate an aortic aneurysm (an insensitive but specific finding) and auscultate the abdomen for any bruits suggestive of vascular disease (e.g. renal artery stenosis and iliac stenosis). Blood on urinalysis may indicate nephritis related to infective endocarditis or a vasculitis (e.g. systemic lupus erythematosis).

chapter 4

Gastrointestinal System

Paul Frankish

General Points

Since the development of imaging modalities such as ultrasound and CT scanning, careful examination of the abdomen is not given the priority it should have in clinical medicine. However, careful examination and sophisticated imaging should be complementary and not interchangeable. Examination does have limitations but a carefully performed examination can yield valuable information and reduce the need for expensive investigations.

It is particularly important when examining the abdomen that the patient is comfortable, warm and as relaxed as possible. The examiner needs to have warm clean hands with well trimmed fingernails and should be gentle in all manoeuvres. Good communication with the patient is essential as this allows the examination to proceed in a logical and timely manner.

The correct positioning of the patient for the examination is important — generally one small pillow under the head provides adequate comfort without causing unwanted contraction of the abdominal muscles. This contraction may inhibit adequate examination of the underlying viscera.

> **Kichu's thoughts . . .**
>
> Practise, Practise, Practise. How long do you have to listen before commenting on bowel sounds.

Apart from the artificial conditions of a viva examination, the abdominal examination is not usually undertaken in isolation. It will generally form part of the general examination with a full history having been already obtained.

Particular note will be taken of how sick the patient appears to be, whether he/she is abnormally pale or pigmented. The state of nutrition and hydration should be observed as well.

> **Kichu's thoughts . . .**
>
> Rectal examination is often not done. Remember the saying that "if you do not put your finger in the rectum, you will put your foot in it."

Peripheral Signs

Diseases of the abdominal organs are associated with a wide array of peripheral signs which should be assiduously searched for. Before you examine the abdomen you should look for the following signs.

Examination of the Hands

In the fingernails, important signs include *leuconychia* or white nails, which is associated with low levels of serum albumin.

Beau's lines are thin pale lines running transversely across the nail coinciding with periods of severe illness or transient hypoalbuminaemia.

Koilonychia or spoon-shaped nails may be found in cases of chronic iron deficiency anaemia.

Finger clubbing is not common in gastrointestinal disease but may occur in chronic liver disease particularly primary biliary cirrhosis and in malabsorptive states such as coeliac disease.

Palmar erythema is redness affecting the periphery of the palms of the hands, particularly the thenar and hypothenar eminences. This is very commonly found in association with alcoholic liver disease. However, it is also found commonly in pregnancy, rheumatoid arthritis and in normal individuals.

Dupuytren's contracture is thickening of the palmar fascia and is associated with alcoholic liver disease. When this condition is severe, patients can develop flexion contractures of the fingers. If the deformity is not obvious, simply stroking your thumb or index finger across the palm will easily reveal the fascial thickening.

CASE STUDY 4.1

A 54-year-old male presents with a one-year history of increasing ankle swelling and abdominal distension. He has a history of heavy alcohol use for many years.

Examination reveals an alert male. He has moderate ascites, hepatomegaly and a 2 cm spleen palpable.

What is the likely diagnosis?
What other signs would you look for in this man?

Examination of the Eyes and Face

The eyes should be examined for evidence of jaundice and inflammation.

Iritis occurs in association with active inflammatory bowel disease. The affected eye is red and painful and there may be decreased visual acuity. With repeated attacks the pupil may become irregular in outline.

Jaundice is generally visible as a yellowish discoloration of the sclera when the total serum bilirubin is >50 μmol/L. As jaundice deepens, the skin becomes yellow and later almost green in severe cholestasis and may be accompanied by skin excoriation due to the associated pruritus.

The tongue should be examined for evidence of *glossitis* with a pale atrophic appearance. An enlarged tongue with peripheral teeth marks may occur where there is macroglossia in some patients with malabsorption.

Asterixis

When liver decompensation occurs, hepatic encephalopathy may ensue. Initially this may involve subtle personality changes with disinhibited behaviour. The patient may then be found to have a

metabolic or flapping tremor, also called *asterixis*. This is demonstrated by having the patient dorsiflex the wrist with the fingers
spread for at least 20 seconds. Flapping tremor consists of intermittent flexion of the fingers as the patient tries to maintain the fingers
in dorsiflexion.

Examination of the Chest

Spider naevi or angiomata are a common finding in chronic liver
disease. They generally but not invariably occur in the distribution
of the drainage area of the superior vena cava, i.e. on the head, upper
chest and arms. They may be a centimetre or more in diameter and
are composed of a central arteriole with radiating capillaries which
blanch on applying pressure to the central arteriole and then refill
from the centre. One or two spider naevi can occur in normal individuals and more in pregnant females but usually more than three is
abnormal.

Breast tissue in a male should be examined for *gynaecomastia*.
After explaining to the patient what you are about to do, gently palpate the subareolar tissue. Usually this is less than 5 mm in diameter
in a male. Feminisation of male hair distribution can occur in chronic
liver disease, with generalised loss of body hair including the male
escutcheon.

The Skin

The skin should be examined for bruising with the presence of
petechiae or *ecchymoses* in malabsorptive states and chronic liver
disease.

Inflammatory conditions of the skin may occur with inflammatory bowel disease. The most common of these are *erythema
nodosum* and *pyoderma gangrenosum*. Erythema nodosum consists of smooth, tender red subcutaneous nodules over the shins.
This is a paniculitis associated most commonly with active
Crohn's disease. Pyoderma gangrenosum is a painless ulcer(s)

which can occur anywhere on the skin. The edge of the ulcer often has bluish discolouration and its appearance may precede the diagnosis of ulcerative colitis. Gluten enteropathy can be associated with *dermatitis herpetiformis*; an intensely itchy blistering rash occurring on the extensor surfaces of the limbs and over the scapulae.

Abdominal Examination

For ease of description, the abdomen may be divided into nine areas or four quadrants as shown in the accompanying diagrams. In the four-quadrant system, imaginary horizontal and vertical lines are drawn through the umbilicus.

Usually for a more precise description of clinical findings, the nine-area method is used. Horizontal lines are drawn at the lower border of the costal margins and the upper borders of the iliac crests and vertical lines through the mid-clavicular lines. This provides nine areas: right and left hypochondria, the epigastrium, right and left flanks, umbilical areas, right and left iliac fossae and suprapubic areas.

The abdomen is then examined in a careful and systematic way. The actual examination performed will be tailored to suit each individual patient.

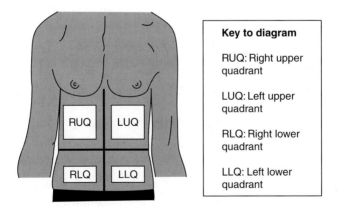

Figure 4.1.   Four Quadrants.

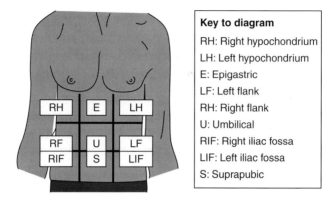

Key to diagram
RH: Right hypochondrium
LH: Left hypochondrium
E: Epigastric
LF: Left flank
RH: Right flank
U: Umbilical
RIF: Right iliac fossa
LIF: Left iliac fossa
S: Suprapubic

Figure 4.2.   Nine Quadrants.

Observation of the Abdomen

Observation of the abdomen is done to detect any abnomal contour due to masses, fluid or enlarged organs. Note should made of any abdominal scars and hernias. The state of the umbilicus should be observed, be it effaced or flattened with ascites or deeply buried in adipose tissue in an obese patient. Dilated superficial veins over the abdomen may be found in portal hypertension. If there is blood flow away from the umbilicus via dilated veins, this is caput medusae, which is rarely seen. Dilated veins over the periphery of the abdomen, with blood flowing cephalad to return to the systemic circulation is a common finding in portal hypertension or inferior vena caval obstruction.

Palpation of the Abdomen

Palpation of the abdomen needs to be gentle and meticulous. It is important to ascertain from the patient whether there is a site of discomfort and to examine this last. Start in one area and then circle the abdomen. Do not forget the umbilical region. It is also appropriate, if there is an obvious mass, to examine the rest of the abdomen first, otherwise other important findings may be missed.

The abdomen should be examined first with light palpation and then with deeper palpation. Remember that palpation is often uncomfortable for the patient so explain what you are doing as you proceed with the examination.

Palpation usually precedes percussion but there are certain circumstances where this rigid pattern should be abandoned. It is much easier to examine the liver and spleen by percussion thereby avoiding patient discomfort with palpation. This will give a good guide to the size of the organs and systematic palpation should start 2 to 3 cm below the area of percussed dullness.

Percussion of the Abdomen

Percussion should be soft within the abdomen as the differences between the solid organs and the bowel in terms of percussion note is often subtle and best elicited with a gentle technique.

In the upper abdomen, the main areas percussed are the liver and spleen. Note that percussion over the kidneys is resonant because they are retroperitoneal with bowel gas anterior to them. This can help you differentiate between an enlarged left kidney and spleen as percussion is dull over the spleen. Dullness over the suprapubic region is usually due to an enlarged bladder. Percussion is a considerate method for testing for abdominal tenderness or peritonism. If gentle percussion yields localised tenderness, this is good evidence for peritoneal irritation and certainly kinder than rebound testing where the palpating fingers are rapidly released from a tender part of the abdomen, generally causing patient undue distress.

Auscultation of the Abdomen

Auscultation generally reveals the presence of bowel sounds. Listen for at least 30 seconds. If you hear no sounds at all, the patient probably has a paralytic ileus. Sounds may be high pitched or tinkling in a mechanical obstruction. Experience will tell you what are normal, increased or reduced bowel sounds.

CASE STUDY 4.2

A 63-year-old female presents with the sudden onset of right upper quadrant pain which radiates posteriorly. Ten years previously, she had been investigated for hepatomegaly and had a CT scan of her liver performed at that time.

She has a strong family history of adult polycystic kidney disease, with six out of seven siblings affected.

What findings would you look for on examination?
What are the likely diagnoses?

Auscultation may reveal bruits in the epigastrium where they are common and often of uncertain significance. Bruits over the liver may occur in association with hepatocellular carcinoma or rarely in alcoholic hepatitis. Over the flanks anteriorly or posteriorly, bruits associated with renal artery stenosis may be heard. Venous hums may be heard over the upper abdomen in patients with portal hypertension. These can be distinguished from arterial bruits in that they tend to be continuous whereas arterial bruits are usually systolic. Venous hums tend to vary in intensity with respiration and the position of the patient.

Assessment of an Abdominal Mass

The assessment of an abdominal mass needs to be done in a systematic fashion. You need to be able to fully describe the special features of abdominal masses and it should include the following features:

- Position (as per the areas above),
- Dimensions — try to accurately measure the surface dimensions,
- Surface characteristics — is it smooth or contoured, how hard is it, is it tender, pulsatile or expansile?

- Is it mobile — does it move with respiration?
- Is there an overlying bruit?

Abdominal masses characteristically occur in specific locations. This knowledge coupled with your careful assessment of the characteristics of the mass should give you important clues as to the nature of the mass.

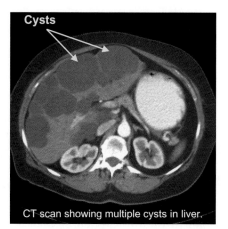

CT scan showing multiple cysts in liver.

Figure 4.3.

Examination of the Liver

The liver is the largest organ in the body but accurate clinical assessment of the precise size of the liver is difficult.

Assessment of a three-dimensional organ by a single potentially unreliable measurement in one dimension is fraught with inaccuracy. It is very important to percuss up and down the abdomen at different sites as livers come in a variety of shapes and sizes. For example, two common variants are the enlarged left lobe of a cirrhotic liver which may be diagnosed as an epigastric mass by the unwary, or the Riedel's lobe variant which is a narrow projection of the right lobe extending down into the right iliac fossa masquerading as gross enlargement of the entire liver.

When palpating the liver, get the patient to take slow, deep breaths and keep your hand still! Let the liver edge come down and meet your fingers. You will miss the liver edge if you are moving your hand when the liver descends on inspiration. You may encounter a markedly enlarged gall bladder in patients with pancreatic cancer or in a mucocele of the gall bladder.

The liver edge that has been percussed out should be examined for tenderness as occurs in acute hepatitis or heart failure, or a hard knobbly liver as in metastatic disease of the liver. The liver may be pulsatile particularly in patients with tricuspid regurgitation and constrictive pericarditis. This is best appreciated by having the patient holding his/her breath in inspiration and feeling for the liver edge with the tips of the fingers. Congested livers are often tender as well. Unfortunately, the assessment of liver consistency, nodularity and even tenderness is unreliable with established liver disease even with expert examiners.

In assessing liver size, the midclavicular line needs to be carefully defined — it is the midpoint of the clavicle between the acromion and the sternum. By convention, the size of the liver is defined by the span in the midclavicular line. The upper border of the liver is usually percussed at about the level of fifth anterior intercostal space. Light percussion should be used from the third space downwards to define the upper border of the liver. If the lower border of the liver cannot be palpated, then the edge is percussed. Percussion alone tends to underestimate the size of the liver because the attenuated thickness of the lower border of the liver may seem resonant to percussion, particularly if it is performed too heavily.

If the distance from the upper border to percussed or preferably palpated liver edge is greater than 13 cm, then genuine hepatomegaly is likely (likelihood ratio 2.5).

Another technique commonly used for assessing liver size is the "scratch test." In this test the diaphragm of the stethoscope is placed at the lower part of the costal margin and while the examiner listens, the abdominal wall is scratched lightly and when scratching is performed over the lower part of the liver, the scratching sound should seem louder. Unfortunately, the correlation between the scratch test and ultrasound assessment of liver size is not good.

Examination for Ascites

Patients with advanced liver disease will commonly have ascites or free intraperitoneal fluid. This may be detected by a number of manoeuvres.

First, observe the patient for bulging of the flanks and effacement of the umbilicus. Next, examine for shifting dullness. This can be done in a number of ways; the objective of which is to show that there is free fluid within the abdominal cavity which will move with gravity. There are two main techniques:

1 Percuss softly from the umbilicus towards the left flank — this avoids percussing over an enlarged liver. Note where the percussion note changes from resonant to dull. At this point you can do one of two things; keep your finger at the site where the percussion note change and roll the patient towards you. If the percussion note is now resonant, you have demonstrated shifting dullness.
2 The second technique is to mark with a ballpoint pen the site of percussion change and then roll the patient away from you and percuss again. If the area of dullness is now closer to the umbilicus, you have demonstrated shifting dullness.

A further technique is the demonstration of a fluid thrill. This requires two examiners. The first examiner places the ulnar surface of his hand vertically up the middle of the abdomen to stop the transmission of soft tissue impulses, while the second examiner flicks one flank with a finger while feeling for a fluid impulse or thrill in the opposite flank.

Ascites is unlikely to be present when the patient does not report any increase in abdominal girth or the patient has no ankle oedema.

There is good observer agreement on the presence of ascites (up to 95%) among a group of senior physicians in one study. The finding of a bulging abdomen, shifting dullness and peripheral oedema makes ascites likely; the converse is also true.

CASE STUDY 4.3

A 58-year-old man presents with a gradual onset of fatigue and breathlessness. He has some vague left upper quadrant discomfort. Examination reveals a massively enlarged spleen extending 20 cm from the left costal margin into the right lower quadrant.

(Continued)

Full blood count reveals a pancytopenia; haemoglobin 76 grams/litre, white cell count 2.8 × 109/L, platelets 62 × 109/L.

Blood film shows immature white blood cells.

What are the likely diagnoses?
What test is likely to be diagnostic?
What further examination findings would you seek?
What further tests may be required?

Examination of the Spleen

Examination of the spleen requires the examiner to palpate from the right iliac fossa up to the left hypochondrium. This part of the examination may be shortened again by percussing first. The spleen is essentially a posterior organ (see attached CT scan) and generally needs to be significantly enlarged before it becomes palpable.

Examination may be easier with the examiner resting the left hand just below the ribs in the left posterior chest and then palpate with the right hand. As with the examination of the liver, you will need to keep the examining hand still as the spleen moves down on inspiration. If you strongly suspect that the spleen should

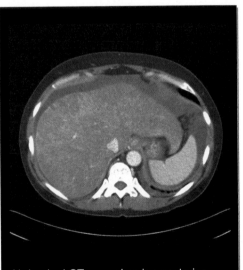

Abdominal CT scan showing posterior position of spleen in a patient with cirrhosis and ascites.

Figure 4.4.

be palpable but you cannot feel it, ask the patient to roll onto his/her right side — this will sometimes make the spleen easier to feel.

Splenic enlargement may be characterised as mild, moderate or massive, with massive spleens such as those found in myelofibrosis or chronic myeloid leukaemia often extending into the right iliac fossa. Big spleens commonly have a palpable "notch" or indentation on the medial aspect. Record the measured distance of the spleen below the left costal margin in the clinical record.

Clinical examination fails to detect splenomegaly in approximately half of the cases. Ultrasound is a very sensitive examination for detection of splenic enlargement and should be undertaken when splenic enlargement is suspected but not found clinically, e.g. a myeloproliferative.

CASE STUDY 4.4

An 80-year-old man presents with intermittent rectal bleeding over a three-month period. He has noticed more frequent bowel action and urgency of defecation. He has a history of prostate cancer treated with radiotherapy five years previously.

Rectal examination reveals a 3 cm mass at the tip of the examining finger which is non-tender and firm.

What is the likely diagnosis?
How would you confirm this?
What further examination findings would you seek?
What further tests may be required?

Rectal Examination

This is a frequently omitted part of the gastrointestinal examination. Sadly, the reluctance to perform a rectal examination can result in inappropriate patient management, e.g. antimotility drugs for overflow incontinence and delays in diagnosis of rectal cancer.

Explain what you are about to do to the patient. Rectal examination is best performed in the left lateral position with the hips flexed to 90 degrees and the legs together. Look for any perianal conditions which may make the procedure painful, e.g. anal fissure or prolapsed piles. Use plenty of lubricant and apply gentle pressure to the sphincters which will relax.

Assessment of sphincter tone is imprecise even by experts but faecal leakage and gaping of the anus when the buttocks are parted suggests a lax sphincter.

Examine all four quadrants and specifically the male prostate for size, contour, consistency and tenderness.

In the female, the cervix is easily palpated anterior to the rectum. Is there any stool in the rectum? After removing the finger, look at the stool on the glove — is there blood, mucus or pus present?

Finally, think of the patient who has just had an unpleasant procedure performed — do not leave them with half a tube of jelly on the perineum and wondering whether or when it will be over! Wipe the area with some tissue and give them some privacy to re-dress, with some more tissue and a bin available if they need it.

Kidney Examination

This is best done for the right kidney with the left hand in the posterior flank and the right hand above it. As the patient takes a deep breath the hands are pushed together and the kidney felt between them. If a kidney is enlarged, it can be balloted (gently bounced) between the two hands.

A normal kidney may be felt in a very thin individual but generally, palpable kidneys are pathologically enlarged.

Note that kidneys are medially sited organs and many people examine too laterally for them (see Fig. 4.3).

Answers to Case Questions

CASE STUDY 4.1

This man has alcoholic liver cirrhosis with evidence of liver failure (ascites).

You would look for signs of chronic liver disease, particularly those of liver decompensation such as jaundice and evidence of a coagulopathy. In this case he is non-encephalopathic but testing of higher mental function and for a flapping tremor would be appropriate.

CASE STUDY 4.2

Look for evidence of liver and kidney enlargement. It is most likely that she has adult polycystic kidney disease with multiple liver cysts.

Pain can occur for a number of reasons with gross hepatomegaly itself causing discomfort. In addition, cysts can become infected or there may be bleeding into the cyst, which is what happened here.

CASE STUDY 4.3

The most likely diagnosis is myelofibrosis but chronic myeloid leukaemia needs to be excluded as do other rarer causes of massive splenomegaly.

A bone marrow examination should be diagnostic.

CASE STUDY 4.4

Rectal cancer or a large rectal polyp would be the most likely diagnosis.

Endoscopic examination and biopsy is required.

Examination should look carefully for any abdominal masses/synchronous lesions and also for liver enlargement/metastatic spread. Further tests would include CT and MRI examinations to accurately stage the tumour.

chapter | 5

The Nervous System: Part I

David Abernethy

Introduction: The Place of Examination in Neurological Problem Solving

---

CASE STUDY 5.1

A 67-year-old right-handed man notices his left arm flops by his side. He tries to tell his wife and she notes slurred but understandable speech. Two hours later he still has hand weakness and dysarthric speech. His wife noticed weakness of the left side of his face.

The clinician thinks "The illness is sudden, and the hand and face are affected as part of the same incident, implying that the problem is much more likely to be in the central nervous system than two lesions, one affecting the facial nerve, another affecting the arm."

"Because it is both sudden," (What) "... and in the CNS," (Where) "...a vascular pathology is most likely, and that is made more likely by his age. Because there is no headache, nausea, vomiting or evolution of new features an infarct is more likely than an intracerebral bleed" (refining "What" still further) "...This is also more likely because the rate of infarct to bleed is about 9:1."

On examination, the visual field is normal. His left mid-face is weak when talking and slightly on showing his teeth. His left hand is weak for finger extension and finger and thumb abduction.

Repetitive finger to thumb apposition is effortful and disproportionately slow. The left arm reflexes are slightly increased. These signs confirm an upper motor neuron lesion affecting his left face and hand. Since the leg is not affected, this is most likely a moderate sized cortical lesion of the right frontal cortex.

The clinician must listen carefully to the history whenever a person's symptoms or signs suggest a neurological problem, or when a third party's reports suggest a neurological problem. (Witness reports are particularly important in the case of behaviour disturbance, communication problems, convulsions, or changes in level of consciousness or cognitive change.)

> **Kichu's thoughts . . .**
>
> The telephone is the most under-utilised medical equipment. When you cannot get a proper history, ring the family or family doctor to get more details.

Early in the history-taking process; it is necessary to establish a complete account of symptoms, other relevant problems and concerns, paying particular attention to their time sequence and duration. Following this, the history will generally take the form of a narrative account by the patient of the onset and evolution of their problems, interrupted by the clinician only to keep the account relevant.

The doctor needs to specify the location on the body, subjective quality, mode of onset and progression over time of each symptom. Very often, careful attention to the very first symptom and its evolution, in the context of the subsequent illness, provides the clue to a difficult problem. It is much more reliable to draw inferences from a patient's spontaneously volunteered description of the evolution of the illness, rather than answers to the clinician's direct questions. Closed questions such as "Did it begin suddenly?" are likely to prompt inaccurate responses that are not reliable.

The aim of the neurological interview is for the clinician to be able to answer two essential questions: "Where is the lesion?" and "What is the lesion?"

"Where" refers to the part of the nervous system affected. The answer may be very anatomically precise (such as "the hand area of the motor cortex"), or may refer to a broader conceptual system (such as "the upper motor neuron pathway affecting voluntary control of the arm").

"What?" refers to the pathological process inferred to have caused the illness. This may initially be expressed in general terms (such as "vascular"), but may be more precisely defined as the diagnostic process progresses such as "a lateral medullary infarction from embolus after vertebral artery dissection".

In many cases, the pathological process can be inferred from the mode of onset of symptoms and their progression. For example, transient and episodic symptoms without long-term damage are commonly caused by migraine or epilepsy. Acute symptoms with persisting damage may be caused by infarction, haemorrhage, trauma, hypoxia or ischaemia. Subacute symptoms that occur over hours, days or weeks may be caused by infection, inflammation, complications of trauma or other acute events and toxicity or deficiency states. Chronic and progressive conditions with worsening of a single symptom or the accumulation of increasing symptoms may be due to tumours, genetic, metabolic and neurodegenerative disease. Chronic but non-progressive conditions may be due to congenital defects or as the results of past infection or trauma.

In practice, the two questions "What?" and "Where?" cannot be completely separated. The answer to one often bears on interpretation of the other. Examination findings will help answer these questions; indeed, they may be critical to confirming or refuting hypotheses generated after analysing the history.

Overview of Neurological Examination: The Four Ps

- Patter — give clear instructions in simple language ("Push to me, pull to you"), with a visual demonstration of what you want the person to do.
- Pattern — follow a stereotyped examination sequence. It is less likely you will forget anything important and with experience, this will allow you to think about the problem while doing the examination. This is particularly useful when you are under pressure or are in an examination.

- Practice — mastery of a professional skill is only acquired by repeated use in the every day task of identifying and solving patient problems. Refection on difficulties and errors with study of areas of identified weakness is needed to develop as a clinician.
- Plan — decide from the problem and history what you need to establish. For example, in a patient with back pain and weak legs of recent onset, upper motor neuron findings will point towards a spinal cord lesion, where absent reflexes and flexor or unresponsive plantars is more suggestive of an acute peripheral neuropathy. This approach will help you realise when you have found signs that alert you that you may have misunderstood the problem and need to rethink your hypothesis. Pay particular attention to the examination findings relevant to the clinical problem.

A 10-Minute Screening and Learning Neurological Examination

Doctors require a systematic, reliable and brief screen of the nervous system that can be carried out quickly with confidence in the results. For detailed discussion of technique, more detailed examination for specific circumstances, interpretation of findings, pitfalls and common abnormalities, see the separate sections devoted to each aspect.

Cranial Nerves

II

Visual acuity: Obtain the best corrected acuity in each eye separately, with glasses or, if needed, a pin hole lens. Use a Snellen Chart at 6 m if available, or a near vision chart. Both are often needed to clarify the state of visual function.

Visual fields: Test by finger movement confrontation for hemi and quadrantic field defects in one or both eyes, including a test for visual neglect with simultaneous movements in both right and left hemifields. When relevant, test the central field to a small ~10 mm red object.

Fundi: Examine the optic disks, including venous pulsation, the adjacent blood vessels and retina.

II and III

Observe: Pupil size and reactions to light and accommodation.

Ptosis: Check the height of the upper eyelid margin position relative to the centre of the pupil.

Saccades and gaze holding/nystagmus: Test the ability to make and sustain voluntary eye movements right, left, up and down.

Pursuit eye movements: Test the ability to pursue a target horizontally to each side.

III, IV and VI

Diplopia: Check eye alignment in the primary and six other lateral cardinal positions (up, horizontal and down on each side) using a target that ensures visual attention and accommodation (draw a large letter "E" on a tongue depressor). Clarify using a cover test if binocular diplopia is reported.

V

Motor jaw opening (check for lateral deviation).

Sensory: Check facial sensation for light touch and pinprick in V1, V2 and V3. This can be combined with the sensory screen towards the end of the examination.

If relevant, test the corneal reflex.

VII

Facial movement: Test movements about the eyes and mouth: eyebrow raising, forcible lid closure, showing teeth, pout, lip closure and filling cheeks while retaining air.

VII

Hearing: Test with a whispered voice in each ear, while masking the other ear by rubbing fingers together. If relevant, examine ear drums.

X

Palate and vocal cord movement: Test soft palate movement on phonation, ask the patient to say "Ah". Ask them to make an explosive cough demonstrating active adduction of both vocal cords.

XI

Trapezius: Shrug shoulders.
Sternomastoid: Rotate head to each side against resistance.

XII

Tongue: Inspection relaxed in the floor of the mouth and on protrusion.

Power testing in arms and legs (including inspection of muscles for wasting and fasciculation)

Weak muscles should be inspected carefully, palpated and compared with the other side. Wasting is especially likely in the first dorsal interosseous, abductor pollicis brevis, tibialis anterior and the small muscles of the feet because these are commonly affected by ulnar, median nerve lesions and peripheral neuropathy respectively.

You will often suspect that the patient is not exerting the maximum power of which they are capable. It is important to vigorously encourage the person. Some muscles can be reliably proven to have normal power objectively by special manoeuvres; see below.
Test the following muscles or movements on every patient:

- Shoulder abduction (external rotation useful in shoulder problems).
- Elbow flexion and extension.

- Wrist flexion and extension (pronation useful if C7 or radial nerve weakness).
- Finger extension, flexion and abduction.
- Thumb abduction in a plane through the index finger and perpendicular to the palm.
- Hip flexion and extension.
- Knee extension and flexion.
- Ankle inversion, dorsiflexion, eversion and plantar flexion.

Other

Test tone in arms and legs for spasticity, hypotonia and, when relevant, for rigidity seen in Parkinsonism (The Guarantors of Brain, 2005).

- Coordination: Finger nose test, heel-shin test, heel-toe (tandem) walking (carefully evaluate eye movements, nystagmus, articulation and alternating hand movements, when relevant).
- Deep tendon reflexes: Biceps, supinator, triceps, knee, ankle and plantar responses.
- Sensation: Ask the patient to outline any area of sensory loss. Screen vibration, position sense, light touch (with eyes closed). Pinprick over face and the dermatomes of the hands and feet, using the distal dorsum of the fingers and toes, just proximal to the nail bed.
- Observe gait and for any movement disorders.

Additional tests

When relevant, it is useful to examine:

- Mental status (an informal assessment is made for each patient during history taking). (Detailed information can be found in (Hodges, 2007) or further reading).
- The ability to swallow.
- The horizontal vestibulo-ocular reflex.
- The Dix–Hallpike test for positional nystagmus.
- The Romberg test.
- The "pull" test for postural reflexes used mainly in Parkinson's and other extrapyramidal syndromes.

Detailed Examination of the Cranial Nerves

Cranial Nerve I: The Olfactory Nerve

Olfaction can be omitted from routine screening examination. Most of the nuances of the flavour of foods are due to olfaction. Loss of taste is very often due to unrecognised loss of the sense of smell. The sense of smell should be tested when patients report loss of taste or smell, in dementia and in unexplained unilateral visual loss (both may be due, rarely, to a frontal meningioma also affecting the olfactory nerve).

Detailed examination technique(s)

Equipment: A (subtle) floral scent is best — coffee, ward soap or perfumed hand cleaner can be used. Don't use a trigeminal irritant such as ammonia, solvent or oil of cloves, since irritants stimulate the fifth nerve pain fibres rather than the sense of smell.

Technique: Test each nostril separately. Ask the patient to close their eyes and report whether they can smell the scent. If they can, ask them to identify it.

Common or important causes of loss of smell

Poor sense of smell without serious cause is common, caused or contributed to by smoking, allergies and ageing. The most important, but rare, pathological cause is a frontal tumour presenting as personality change, self neglect, depression and apathy. Sometimes such people have been thought, unfortunately, to be depressed or demented over months to years.

- Sudden onset: Head injury (usually permanent).
- Subacute onset: Post-viral infection such as a severe cold or flu (can be permanent).
- Multiple sclerosis.

- Chemotherapy — the olfactory neurons are the only neurons known to undergo cell division which may contribute to their vulnerability.
- Insidious onset: Alzheimer's disease, Parkinson's disease, temporal arteritis and chronic meningitis, such as sarcoidosis.

Cranial Nerve II: The Optic Nerve

Screening when there is no reason to suspect a lesion

- Test visual (VA) acuity in each eye, without and with, best correction, glasses, lenses or a pinhole.
- Examine the fundi, including the optic disks, adjacent retinal vessels and background, including the macula.
- Test visual fields in each eye separately to confrontation with a moving finger. Test the upper nasal and temporal fields separately to exclude first a field defect, then simultaneously to exclude hemi-neglect. Then repeat for the lower quadrants.
- Test pupil reactions to light.

The purpose of testing visual acuity in the context of neurological illness is to establish normal retinal, optic nerve and visual pathway function. Refractive error is not relevant to neurological diagnosis except as a complicating difficulty.

The ability to discriminate colour, particularly red, is impaired earlier and to a greater degree in optic nerve disease and is a more sensitive test of optic nerve function than acuity. This is the basis of the use of red objects to detect subtle areas of visual field loss.

Equipment for VA testing: VA is best tested with a Snellen Chart at 6-metre distance, precisely measured. Adequate illumination is required. Alternatively, use a near vision chart at a standard reading distance of 35 cm.

Many patients have poor acuity from refractive error at only distance or only near so that testing both at distance and near is useful in practice if one or other is abnormal. Patients over 45 often have presbyopia and often have not brought reading glasses. Refractive error can be excluded as cause of the impaired acuity under this and other circumstances using a pinhole as a lens. Use a safety pin to make about six large ~1 mm holes arranged in a 1 cm diameter circle in a piece of card.

Technique: Test each eye in turn without, then with glasses. If the patient has spectacles, cover one eye with an occluder or with cotton wool behind the lens. Use finger counting in central vision at 1 metre then perception of light as measures of acuity if it is very poor.

Colour vision

As a simple effective screening test for unilateral loss of colour perception, ask the person to compare the colour of a red object centrally in each eye. Pink, yellow brown or black may be reported from affected areas of the visual field. Formal testing requires Ishihara isochromatic test plates or similar. These are often only available in Neurology or Eye departments.

How to examine the fundi

The patient is asked to look at, or imagine they are looking at, a fixed distant point. The examiner looks through the opthalmoscope first at the light beam on own hand through the ophthalmoscope, then moves the light beam to the patient's eye at about 15 degrees temporal to the patient's line of fixation. Move closer to the patient's eye along this line. You should now be looking at or near to the optic disk. Work back along retinal vessels to the disk if necessary.

Retinal abnormalities you should learn to recognise

- Venous pulsation on the optic disk: Indicative of normal CSF pressure (although this is often absent in about 40% of persons with normal CSF pressure).
- Papilloedema: Optic nerve axon flow obstruction from raised CSF pressure causes a swollen disk without visual loss.

- Papillitis: Optic nerve inflammation or infarction causes a swollen disk with visual loss (poor acuity).
- Diabetic retinopathy.
- Hypertensive retinopathy.

Visual fields (Fig. 5.1)

Test each eye separately. Begin (one eye at a time) by asking the person to look at your face. Ask successively "Can you see my face? Can you see both sides? Is there any difference between the two sides?" Then hold up two hands, one in each of the upper quadrants. Ask "How many hands can you see?" Avoid the leading question "Can you see two hands?" Repeat this in the lower quadrants. The person with a field defect may see only one hand, or if they see two, may report that one is blurred or indistinct.

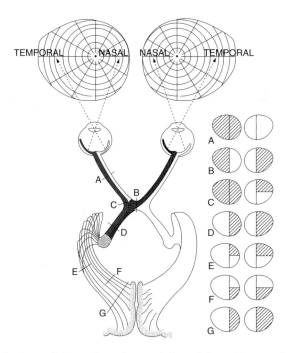

Figure 5.1. Lesions of the optic pathways (adapted from Homans (1940)).

When you are testing visual fields, have the patient fixate on your nose and only perform the test movements when you can see this is the case. Persons with field defects rapidly realise they are not seeing some targets and will subconsciously anticipate and move their eyes to detect your test movements.

Visual field defects are often not areas of absolute blindness and may be subtle. They also may recover gradually after acute stroke. Large movements may be detected in areas of relative field loss. Therefore, finger movements used for field testing should be made with a single finger and be of small amplitude — approximately 1 cm.

Use small finger movements from both hands as two alternative targets. Test one quadrant against the other, lower right against lower left, upper right against upper left. Randomise presentation of testing movements in each side of the field. If you find a defect, check the vertical and horizontal meridians carefully. Do this by moving the hand in the blind field progressively closer to the boundary of interest between presentations of finger movement. Make most of the test movements in the normal field so the patient does not know when to expect a stimulus in the "blind" field.

As with any sensory defect, test from any area of lost vision towards an area in which the person can see normally. Having the patient count the number of fingers, 1, 2 or 5, that you display in each quadrant can be an effective and rapid means of confirming a subtle field defect.

Common and important field defects

Homonymous hemianopsia or quadrantanopia is, in most cases, due to lesions in the optic radiation or in the occipital cortex. A defect will affect either the same hemi-fields or the same quadrants in both eyes.

An occipital cortex lesion may show macula sparing. This can be demonstrated if a confrontation stimulus is seen sooner as it approaches the vertical meridian from the blind field along the horizontal meridian, compared with a target brought along a parallel path in the upper or lower field.

Optic nerve and chiasmal lesions cause areas of loss of sensitivity to red long before there is loss of sensitivity to black on white (tested by the visual acuity test). In an optic nerve lesion, a red pin may lose its colour and appear dull or "desaturated". This is referred to as a relative rather than an absolute scotoma (a blind spot).

A central scotoma usually results from optic nerve disease, but may also be seen in macular disease. It produces a central blind area to red, with a peripheral zone in which a red object can be seen. Patients with optic nerve disease of moderate or severe degree often also with a relative afferent pupillary defect.

Bitemporal hemianopia is almost invariably due to lesions of the optic chiasm. As lesions in the region of the chiasm first affect fibres supplying the nasal retina, patients have a defect of vision in their temporal field. Pituitary tumours are the commonest cause, in which case the upper temporal field in one eye is typically affected first. Craniopharyngiomas and aneurysms are a much less common cause. These defects are usually subtle.

Retinal fibre bundle defects (such as occur in glaucoma) may produce a "nasal step". Use the index fingers of each hand, one above and one below the horizontal meridian brought from the nasal periphery towards the point of fixation. Check if they can see one or two fingers as they first become visible.

Common or important causes of lesions of the optic nerve

Optic neuritis

Optic neuritis is more common in women and commonly affects the 18 to 40 years age group. Typical history and symptoms include pain on movement of the eye, with a fog or patch in front of the eye (central vision), particularly affecting colours (which look washed out). Vision worsens over hours to a few days, sometimes to complete blindness. It remains poor for several weeks and then gradually improves over 4–6 weeks, although often not completely. There may be papilloedema, but often no abnormality of the optic fundus (depending on the location of the lesion in the nerve). Depth perception may be impaired and there is usually an afferent pupillary defect in severe cases. Later temporal or diffuse optic disk pallor may occur from axon loss and reduced metabolic demand for capillary flow on the disk.

Anterior ischaemic optic neuropathy

Sudden painless unilateral visual loss in an older person, typically over 60 years is a characteristic presentation. There is usually severe impairment of visual acuity which seldom improves. The field defect is an upper or lower altitudinal scotoma with involvement of central vision. There is pale swelling of the disc with a few linear haemorrhages. Infarction of the optic nerve head results from occlusion of the posterior ciliary arterioles. More than 20% of cases are due to

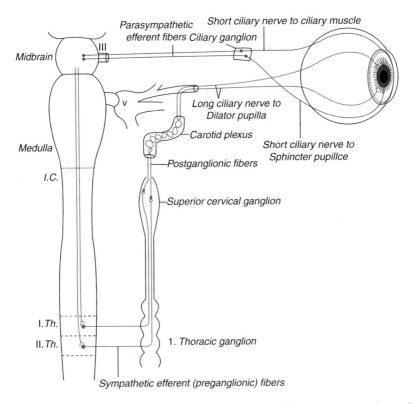

Figure 5.2. Sympathetic connections of the ciliary and superior cervical ganglia (adapted from Gray (1918)).

temporal arteritis, with high risk of visual loss in the other eye and of posterior circulation stroke in the arteritic form.

Compressive optic neuropathy

This rare but important condition produces an insidious loss of central, especially colour vision, in one eye. This may be noticed suddenly, such as when the other eye is closed for some reason, e.g. from water or grit. The usual cause is meningioma of the optic nerve sheath which may sometimes be difficult to visualise on MRI. As a general rule, insidious loss of function in any single nervous structure suggests compression by tumour.

Pupil size

Pupil size in persons without neurological or ocular disease reflects the balance of the relative sympathetic and parasympathetic tone, ambient light, ocular accommodation, some drugs and is also affected by age (older persons have smaller pupils). In a person with severe midbrain damage, for instance after compression from diffuse brain swelling or irretrievable brain death with no cerebral circulation, the pupils are about 5 mm in diameter and have subtle irregularity of outline — reflecting complete relaxation.

Pupil constriction to light is an active parasympathetic reflex. Pupil dilatation in the dark beyond 5 mm (mid-position) is an active sympathetic reflex. The afferent input is from the optic nerve with axons stimulating the Edinger–Westphal nuclei.

Parasympathetic fibres of the efferent pathway are carried in both third nerves, reaching the pupil via the ciliary nerves.

Horner's syndrome

Lesions to the sympathetic pathways that enervate the pupil cause Horner's syndrome (which consists of the triad of miosis, ptosis and anhydrosis on the affected side of the face). The sympathetic part of the efferent pathway has three conceptually separate components (a central section, the pre-ganglionic fibres and the post-ganglionic fibres) that can be distinguished clinically.

The central section extends from the hypothalamus, down the ipsilateral brain stem and lateral spinal cord to the ciliospinal centre at C8-T1. Lesions of the brainstem or spinal cord that affect this pathway cause loss of sweating of the whole of that half of the face and body.

The pre-ganglionic fibres for the head and neck are part of the T1 and T2 roots, travel over the lung apex, thence via the sympathetic chain to synapse in the superior cervical ganglion. A common lesion in this pathway occurs from apical lung carcinomas, which may also affect nerves to the arm (causing Pancoast's syndrome).

Post-ganglionic fibres travel in the sheath of the common carotid. Fibres to the pupil are carried to the eye on the internal carotid and its branches. Carotid artery dissection is an important cause of lesions in this section of the pathway. The presence of facial sweating suggests the lesion is above the carotid bifurcation since the sweat fibres separate and reach the face along branches of the external carotid artery.

In Horner's syndrome, the disparity in pupil size is more apparent in the dark and after a loud noise (both of which activate the sympathetic pupil dilator fibres). The pupil involvement can be confirmed and distinguished from physiological anisocoria by confirming slowness of and reduced amplitude of dilatation of the affected pupil in the dark. An infrared video camera is very useful.

Pharmacological tests are widely recommended to confirm and localise the lesion in Horner's syndrome. These tests are impractical outside of specialised ophthalmology clinics (Danesh-Meyer et al., 2004).

Pupil size and reaction to light is the single most valuable piece of information in the evaluation of the person in a coma and if normal, almost always indicates a drug-induced, metabolic or diffuse brain dysfunction as the cause.

Testing the pupils and eyelids

Examine:

- Eyelid position
- Pupil size, equality and regularity

- Reactions to light and to dark
- Reaction to accommodation

To examine ptosis, check the upper eyelid position in relation to the centre of the pupil (mid-corneal reflex) in the primary position. This should be at least 2 mm and there should be no more than 2 mm difference between the two lids.

The upper lid margin excursion should be 12–17 mm from extreme up to down gaze, this is useful to distinguish levator dehiscence (excursion normal) from neurologic causes, in which it is reduced (Miller *et al.*, 2008).

Pupil light reaction

When possible and particularly when this is an important issue, examine the patient in dim light. Use magnification when needed, cheap three dioptre spectacles are very useful, the auroscope lens or the ophthalmoscope focused on the pupil are all effective. A very bright light is needed. This is especially important in comatose patients, who generally have small pupils, in which the magnitude of reaction is reduced but is a critical discriminator of the likely cause of coma.

Afferent pupillary defect

Test when there is unexplained unilateral or asymmetric loss of visual acuity, or colour vision loss, suggesting possible optic nerve disease (the afferent pathway of the pupillary light reflex). When the affected eye is directly stimulated with light, the pupillary reaction is less complete compared to the consensual pupil constriction achieved in the same eye by stimulating the opposite eye.

Thus, when swinging a flashlight from the normal to the affected eye, instead of dilating slightly during the movement of the light and then constricting again as the eye is directly stimulated, the pupil of the affected eye continues to dilate while the light is shining on it.

An afferent pupillary defect is seen with an optic nerve lesion and may also occur with extensive, obvious, central retinal disease. In normal light, the pupils are equal, except in their direct and consensual responses.

Accommodation

This is best achieved using a distant target and the patient's own thumb. Dim light helps, because the pupil will be less constricted and the effect of accommodation on pupil diameter more apparent.

Common or important causes of pupil or lid abnormalities

Physiological anisocoria (difference in pupil size) is reported in 20% of normal people in dim light — although there is usually only about 0.4 mm disparity. It is seen in 10% of people in room light and is usually less than 0.6 mm, but can be up to 1.0 mm.

Levator dehiscence due to aging or damage to the upper lid, levator palpebrae superioris or its aponeurosis may also cause ptosis without papillary change.

In myasthenia gravis, there is upper lid fatigue which may be demonstrated by 60 seconds sustained upgaze. This is not specific but highly suggestive. There are usually other typical features including variable diplopia and weakness of orbicularis oculi. Muscular dystrophies, such as myotonic dystrophy, may also cause bilateral ptosis, as may mitochondrial myopathies.

Adie's pupil

Adie's pupil is a common abnormality in which the pupil is typically large when first noticed (although later in the progression of the condition becomes smaller) and does not react, or reacts sluggishly to light, but constricts and dilates slowly in response to accommodation. Adie's pupil is often associated with depressed tendon reflexes. Patients may complain about slowness to adapt to bright lights.

Argyll Robertson pupils

Argyll Robertson pupils are a rare consequence of syphilis, in which pupils are small, irregular and unreactive to light but react normally to accommodation. They may be associated with absence of position sense, deep pain and ankle jerks, with up-going toes.

Cranial Nerves III, IV and VI: The Optic, Oculomotor and Trochlear Nerves

Disorders of eye movements may be conceptualised as supranuclear or internuclear, nuclear or infranuclear. Supranuclear lesions are analogous to upper motor lesions in the peripheries, while nuclear and infranuclear lesions are analogous to lower motor neuron motor weakness.

Supranuclear disorders occur with lesions in brain pathways responsible for coordinated movement of the eyes. Nuclear or infranuclear lesions affect the lower motor neuron pathway, in the nerve either within or outside the CNS, the neuromuscular junction or the muscle. There are important practical problems at each site encountered relatively often in internal medicine and neurology.

Diplopia

The brain receives no direct feedback from eye muscles and relies on the position of the image of the object of interest on the retina in relation to the fovea to project it in space. The assumption made by the brain in locating the object in space, relative to the intended point of fixation, is that the eyes are correctly aligned. If one eye is deviated towards the nose, (esotropia) the object of interest is seen with the fovea of the fixing eye, but its image is displaced horizontally on to the nasal retina of the deviated eye. This "false" image is projected by the brain in space as if both eyes are fixing on the same point. Thus the false image is projected temporally to the true image, producing diplopia. The same principles apply to projection of vertical and torsional separation of true and false images.

Terminology of eye movements

- **Primary position:** Eyes looking at a distant target straight ahead, at level.
- **Cardinal positions of gaze:** Primary, up, down, right, left, up and down to right and to left respectively.
- **-tropia:** A manifest ocular misalignment, i.e. the eye, although directed by the brain at the target, is deviated.

- **-phoria:** Deviation present only if binocular fusion is interrupted (usually by the cover/uncover or alternate cover test).
- **Cover test:** A simple technique to demonstrate whether or not an eye is fixing on the target, by covering the other eye and looking closely for a "movement of redress" as the deviated eye takes up fixation. The test establishes whether or not there is a tropia. If this is the paretic eye, this is the primary deviation.
- **Cover/uncover test:** Observes the behaviour of the covered eye as the cover is removed. If there is no tropia, this test will detect any phoria.
- **Alternate cover test:** In paralytic strabismus, allows demonstration of which eye has the primary (smaller) and secondary (larger) deviation.
- **Comitant deviation:** Deviation to the same degree in all positions of gaze, seen in childhood strabismus and in long standing paralytic strabismus due to adaptive alteration in muscle activation.
- **Incomitant deviation:** Ocular misalignment which varies with the direction of gaze.
- **Saccades:** Voluntary eye movements to a target.
- **Pursuit eye movements:** Involuntary smooth tracking movements of a slowly moving target.

Patients with the new onset of ocular misalignment typically report diplopia. Less commonly, the patient notices visual confusion instead, as the consequence of different images seen simultaneously at the fovea of both eyes. Some patients with a mild disparity may notice blurred vision that disappears when either eye is covered.

Not all patients with misalignment report diplopia. Diplopia is absent in patients who have experienced squint since childhood. These patients often have misalignment that is the same in all directions of gaze, referred to as comitant.

New onset diplopia is usually worse with a gaze in one direction, typically into the field of gaze of the weak muscle. Usually, the person will fixate with the unaffected/non-paretic eye; however, the ability to alternate fixation may make the patient's report of the distance between images confusing. Careful objective testing using the cover, cover uncover and alternate cover tests will resolve the cause.

Primary and secondary deviations

The eye muscles function as yoked pairs to move both eyes to fixate on the same point in space. For example, the yoked pairs when looking horizontally to the right are the left medial rectus and the right lateral rectus; looking down while looking right involves the left superior oblique and right inferior rectus; while looking up and right involves the left inferior oblique and the right superior rectus.

To force a weak muscle of the yoke pair to take up fixation requires a larger innervation to both members of the pair. This results in a greater (secondary) deviation of the normal than the paretic eye. This is the basis of the cover, cover–uncover and alternate cover tests.

For example, in the case of a partial right sixth nerve palsy, while looking right, both the left medial rectus and right lateral rectus must contract. Both muscles receive identical innervation (Hering's law). When fixing with the normal left eye an object to the right of the primary position — a position where the paretic right eye is still capable of fixation — the right eye will be deviated slightly nasally (the primary deviation). If the right eye is then forced to fixate the same object by covering the left eye, greater innervation to both members of the yoke pair will be needed to move the right eye into position. This causes the left eye to deviate to a greater degree behind the cover (the secondary deviation). Provided the patient does not have other problems, the alternate cover test will determine which deviation is primary and secondary for the affected yoke pair.

Evaluation of the patient with diplopia

Examine and record the movement of each eye alone (ductions) and then both together in each of the nine cardinal positions of gaze. Perform this examination with the patient fixating both at near and at distance, ideally 6 metres. This is especially important for sixth nerve palsy, which may be better detected at distance, since less lateral rectus contraction is required to fixate during accommodation. Testing with a 6 metre fixation target also helps to exclude physiological diplopia (when the short focal distance may lead the patient to report irrelevant and misleading physiological diplopia).

Use a target with visual interest (such as a letter or a small picture on a tongue depressor) and watch the pupils as a guide to accommodation (dilatation may imply looking into the distance rather than at the target).

Perform a cover test in each of the nine cardinal positions of gaze. Use one distant target, such as a letter on a Snellen chart, positioning the patient's head. During the cover test observe for movement as the deviated contralateral eye takes up fixation. If the cover test is negative but one eye deviates behind the cover (cover/uncover test), there is a phoria or latent deviation.

If there is a manifest deviation in one or more directions, use the alternate cover test to establish the primary and secondary deviation. This can be used to determine which muscle is paretic.

Saccades

Saccades are fast eye movements made to shift fixation to a particular point in space. Saccadic abnormalities are common in stroke, demyelination and cerebellar disease. Saccades may have delayed initiation and or are slowed in many chronic degenerative brain diseases.

If saccades clearly overshoot (hypermetric) or undershoot the target (hypometric), requiring an extra movement to fixate on it, this is a distinctive feature of cerebellar disease.

Supranuclear and internuclear eye movement disorders

Supranuclear lesions may cause gaze paralysis, with the patient unable to look in one direction: up, down or to one side. Horizontal and vertical vestibulo-ocular reflexes can be used to demonstrate whether or not the nuclear, internuclear and lower motor neuron components are intact.

Internuclear ophthalmoplegia

Internuclear ophthalmoplegia results from a unilateral lesion of the median longitudinal fasciculus (MLF) rostral to the sixth nerve nucleus. There is slowness and, in more severe lesions, weakness or complete paralysis of adduction of the ipsilateral medial rectus and large amplitude "ataxic" nystagmus of the contralateral eye on gaze to the opposite side, beating to that side. When the lesion also involves the sixth nerve nucleus, a "one and a half" syndrome of inability to look to the ipsilateral side and on looking to the contralateral side, only that eye abducts (no horizontal movement of the ipsilateral eye).

Causes of eye movement abnormality

Myasthenia gravis

Myasthenia produces weakness of eyelid opening (ptosis), of eyelid closure (orbicularis oculi) and of individual extraocular muscles. It is characteristically variable and can mimic any extraocular weakness, including an internuclear ophthalmoplegia.

The weakness of myasthenia is improved for at least a few minutes after sleep and worsens as the day goes on. It also worsens with use of the muscle. Fatigue can be demonstrated by sustained upgaze for 60 seconds.

There are several interesting phenomena highly suggestive of myasthenia:

1. Cogan's lid twitch sign — on looking down for 20 seconds then up, the eyelid(s) momentarily rises then falls and may twitch several times.
2. Increase in ptosis of one eyelid on passive elevation of the other lid.

Thyroid eye disease

This is a feature of Graves disease (autoimmune thyroid disease), but may occur when there is no disturbance of thyroid function. There is typically proptosis, lid lag and restriction of eye muscles, most often the inferior and medial recti. The main differential diagnosis is orbital lymphoma and orbital pseudotumour (a non-specific inflammatory disorder).

Nystagmus

Nystagmus is a disorder of fixation. The underlying abnormality in nystagmus is a slow drift of the eyes away from steady fixation. In "jerk nystagmus", these slow movements are followed by a rapid corrective eye movements. In the less common pendular nystagmus, the refixations are also slow. Vision is affected if the image slips off the fovea and is less clear the further it slips into the peripheral retina during the slow phase. This can cause either blurring or a perception of movement of the image, oscillopsia. There is no perception of movement during the fast refixations.

Jerk nystagmus is named for the position in which it is seen and for the direction of the quick phases. Nystagmus, in which the fast movement is to the left and which is seen only on left gaze, is referred to as first-degree, left beating nystagmus. If it is also evident in the primary position, it is second-degree. If left beating nystagmus is still seen even while looking right, it is referred to as third-degree. Alexander's Law states that nystagmus is most severe with gaze in the direction of the quick phases.

End-point nystagmus may be seen in normal people on extremes of eccentric gaze. It may be asymmetrical, but is poorly sustained and there is no rebound.

Gaze-evoked nystagmus occurs only when the eyes are moved away from the primary position. If the position is sustained the nystagmus may diminish. When the eyes are returned to the primary position, a brief nystagmus beating in the opposite direction — rebound nystagmus — may occur. Alcohol, sedatives and anticonvulsant intoxication are the most common causes, and it may also be typically seen in cerebellar disease.

Peripheral causes of nystagmus are discussed below (under Cranial Nerve VIII) and further reading and video examples can be found in "The neurology of eye movements" (Leigh *et al.*, 2006).

Cranial Nerve V: The Trigeminal Nerve

The fifth cranial nerve (the trigeminal nerve) provides sensation to the face, inside the mouth, the anterior 2/3 of the tongue and the motor supply to the muscles of mastication: masseter, temporalis and the pterygoids.

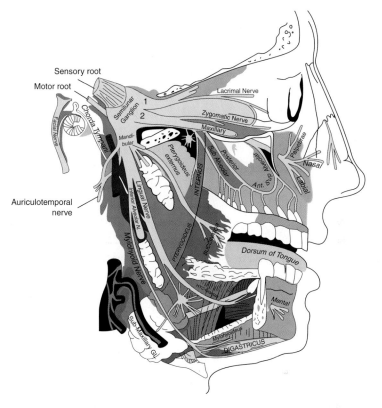

Figure 5.3.   Distribution of the maxillary and mandibular nerves and the submaxillary ganglion (adapted from Gray (1918)).

Light touch fibres from the trigeminal nerve carry touch sensation to the principal sensory nucleus in the mid pons, cross the brainstem to the medial lemniscus and ascend to the thalamus. Pain and temperature sensation from the face is conveyed to the contralateral thalamus via the descending nucleus of the fifth nerve which extends from the mid pons to C1 or C2. The corneal response is also carried via this nucleus and can be affected by pressure on the brainstem from a cerebellopontine angle lesion.

Fibres from the periphery of the face descend most caudally in an onion like pattern. Syringomyelic cavities in the central spinal cord, usually extending upwards from the cervical enlargement, gradually and progressively damage these fibres from below, causing a balaclava helmet pattern of sensory loss to pain and temperature.

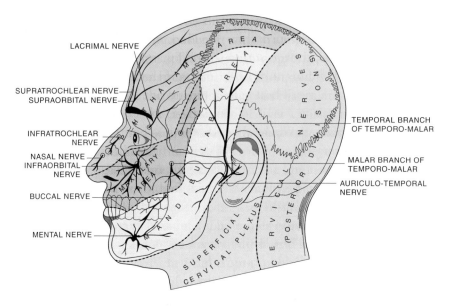

Figure 5.4.   Sensory areas of the head, showing the general distribution of the three divisions of the fifth nerve (adapted from Gray (1918)).

Examination of the trigeminal nerve

Facial numbness is common in trigeminal nerve lesions whereas jaw weakness is very unusual.

To test facial sensation, use light touch and pin prick to each side of the mid line over the forehead, maxilla, upper lip and chin. If reduced sensation is reported, establish its boundaries in relation to the distribution of the divisions of the fifth nerve and the midline. Usually this means testing medially, laterally, up and down until the stimulus is reported normal, paying attention to the known boundaries of the three divisions of the fifth nerve.

Functional face numbness is common, but attention to the boundaries of the trigeminal innervation, particularly over the angle of the jaw and in the hair near the vertex, is helpful in discriminating organic sensory loss.

The corneal reflex

Test the corneal response with a wisp of cotton wool carefully twisted to avoid loose fibres that may inadvertently touch other structures, such as the lashes or conjuctiva. Explain what you are about to do. Ask the patient to look up slightly to expose as much cornea as possible. Approach the cornea from the side. Lightly touch the lateral cornea below the pupil to avoid provoking a visual reflex blink.

A normal response to the corneal reflex is a blink of both eyes. Some patients have very insensitive corneas and little or no response. In this situation, check if the stimulus can be felt. This information is less reliable.

Ptosis

A droopy lid and large pupil that does not react to light is likely to be caused by a third nerve palsy. The eye will also be turned down and out with diplopia. The usual cause is an aneurysm on the posterior communicating artery.

If there is a painless third nerve palsy and the pupil is not involved, the likely cause is diabetic or hypertensive small vessel disease.

Ptosis without pupil change may be idiopathic or congenital or related to squint. Unilateral or bilateral ptosis may occur with acute unilateral hemisphere lesions, but this is rare. Midbrain lesions involving the third nerve nucleus cause bilateral ptosis, since the nucleus for the eyelids is the midline.

Testing the motor function of the trigeminal nerve

Palpate the temporalis and masseter muscles as the person clenches their jaw.

Unilateral pterygoid weakness causes jaw deviation to that side, and weakness can be confirmed by lateral pressure on the partially open jaw. Jaw deviation alone is seldom a relevant observation if detected in routine exam of an asymptomatic patient.

The jaw jerk

Ask the person to open their mouth partially, so that the jaw is not tense. Rest your finger on their jaw below their lower lip and tap on

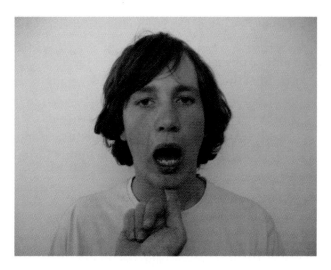

Figure 5.5.   Pterygoid weakness causes jaw deviation towards the weak side.

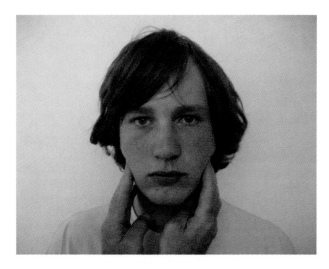

Figure 5.6.   Masseters.

your finger with the tendon hammer. The jaw jerk is often absent in normals.

The jaw jerk is exaggerated in upper motor neuron lesions above the mid pons and is seen in bilateral pyramidal tract lesions of any cause. It can be helpful evidence of a lesion above the cervical spine in suspected motor neurone disease.

An exaggerated jaw jerk is sometimes accompanied by emotional lability, slow effortful "spastic" speech (Have the patient repeat "La La La" as quickly as possible. Spastic dysarthria produces "Laa... Laa... Laa...") and difficulty swallowing. This is referred to as a pseudobulbar palsy and is most commonly a sign of bilateral cerebrovascular disease. Some normal people have very brisk reflexes, including the jaw jerk.

Loss of trigeminal sensation

Sensory loss for touch and pain over the whole territory of the nerve implies a lesion of the ganglion or of the sensory root. Individual divisions can be affected in lesions of the cavernous sinus or of the orbital fissure, often associated with diplopia. Loss of touch only (and not pain) may occur from a lesion of the main sensory nucleus in the pons. Loss of pain and temperature only occurs with lesions involving the descending tract, nucleus or ascending tracts at any level of the brainstem below the mid pons and is more common.

Idiopathic trigeminal neuropathies are not unusual and are presumably either viral or inflammatory. Onset is over days, followed by a plateau for several weeks, with gradual slow recovery. They are often associated with hypersensitivity. Some are associated with connective tissue diseases particularly Sjogren's syndrome and these do not generally recover.

Facial pain

Pain in the face is very common. Trigeminal neuralgia is a specific syndrome of momentary severe shooting pains in one division of the fifth nerve (most commonly V3 or less often V2) without sensory loss. Pain is often set off by sensory stimuli of touching, cold air, chewing or speaking and commonly responds to antiepileptics such as carbemazepine.

Unilateral localised facial pain followed by progressive sensory loss in one division suggests malignant infiltration, possibly by perineurial invasion of subcutaneous branches by a squamous cell tumour, which may not be obvious on the skin.

Cranial Nerve VII: The Facial Nerve

Voluntary movement of one side of the face is controlled by the contralateral cerebral motor cortex, via the pyramidal tract to the facial nerve nucleus (similar to control of the limbs). The facial nerve nucleus also receives significant input from the ipsilateral pyramidal tract. This is more marked for upper face movements which rarely appear weak after hemiparesis.

Voluntary and emotional control of facial expression by the brain

Emotional responses, e.g. for smiling or laughing, are conveyed by a separate pathway possibly originating in the limbic system, so that after a lateral hemisphere lesion causing facial weakness, movements evoked by emotional stimuli may be more rapid and complete. (This is why it is important to avoid amusing the patient during tests of voluntary facial movement.)

The facial nerve supplies only one side of the face so that a complete lower motor neuron lesion causes complete paralysis of all muscles of facial expression on that side of the face. There are a wide range of possible sites of a lower motor neuron lesion and accurate localisation of the site of the lesion is a strong clue to the pathological process (see below). Localisation is often possible by considering information from the history about the involvement of taste, tears and the nerve to Stapedius — involvement of which causes hyperacusis. It is especially important to consider involvement of the facial nerve in the parotid gland if the lesion is purely motor, particularly if it is progressive.

Careful documentation of the degree weakness of each move-ment is prudent at the initial and subsequent visits. Digital photography, with appropriate consent, can be very helpful to assess change over time.

Examination of the facial nerve

Watching mid-facial movement during the interview is the most sensitive way to detect the typical flattening and reduced movement of the upper lip typical of a subtle upper motor neuron lesion. Vigorous eye closure and showing teeth without causing laughter is sufficient to exclude LMN lesion.

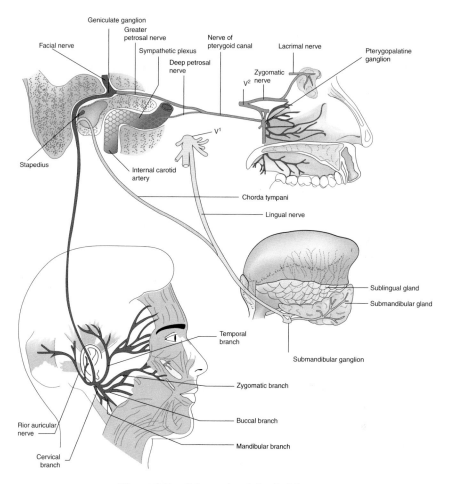

Figure 5.7. Schematic of the facial nerve.

Careful testing of the following range of movements will give a comprehensive view of function, allow a decision about any degree of or region of weakness and can be performed quickly.

- Eyebrow raising and frowning — check symmetry and for forehead wrinkling.
- Eye closure — check that the lashes are almost buried (although persons wearing contact lenses or makeup may be reluctant to fully exert themselves). In unilateral severe weakness, the eye does not close but the eyeball rolls upward — Bell's phenomenon.

- Snarling.
- Teeth showing, lip pursing, forcible lip closure.
- Platysma contraction.
- Ask the patient to puff their cheeks with lips closed and test the ability to retain air to light simultaneous pressure on both cheeks. This may reveal unilateral orbicularis oris weakness.
- Inspect the middle ear, test hearing and palpate the parotid if relevant.

Testing taste is difficult using the classical sweet, sour, salt and bitter stimuli. The results are often ambiguous and as a result, not diagnostically helpful.

Common or important causes of lesions

Lower motor neuron lesions

As with any cranial nerve, a lesion may occur in the brainstem, subarachnoid space, meninges, skull base or during its extracranial course.

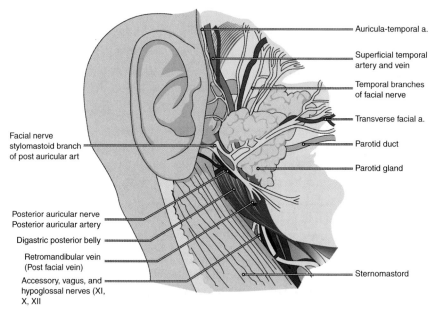

Figure 5.8.   The relation between the facial nerve and parotid gland.

Bell's palsy is the most frequently recognised idiopathic cranial mononeuropathy. The mode of onset, associated hyperacusis and loss of taste help to distinguish distal lesions, which are relatively rare but often due to involvement by parotid malignancy.

The Ramsay Hunt syndrome (due to herpes zoster) causes pain in the ear, and vesicles in the ear canal and on the soft palate. It otherwise resembles Bell's palsy.

There are a large number of other potential causes of facial nerve lesions or facial weakness, most of which are unusual or rare. The facial nucleus or fascicle may be involved in any lesion of the lateral pons. Basal meningitis from sarcoidosis and other forms of chronic meningitides such as Lyme disease or tuberculosis may also cause facial palsy, as may malignant meningitis from carcinoma or lymphoma. Otitis media is a possible but rare cause in the western world. Squamous cell carcinoma of the skin may infiltrate individual fascicles producing a gradual increase in localised paralysis.

Other disorders

"Hemifacial spasm" is a relatively common movement disorder in the middle aged and elderly. There are repeated fine jerking movements about the eye and corner of the mouth that may be due to irritation of the nerve by a vascular loop in the posterior fossa.

"Myokymia" is a fine continuous rippling, undulating movement of facial muscles seen in MS, with demyelinating neuropathy and brainstem tumours.

Aberrant regeneration of the facial nerve may cause "synkinetic movements" in which, for example, blinking the eye may lead to contraction around the mouth.

Cranial Nerve VIII: The Vestibulocochlear Nerve (Or "Acoustic Nerve" Or "Cochlear Nerve")

The ear has two functional parts, a system for conducting and amplifying sound and a system for perceiving sound. There are two clinically distinguishable types of deafness. Conductive deafness is caused by processes that affect the conducting/amplifying system,

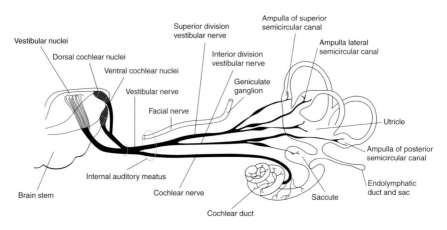

Figure 5.9. Schematic diagram of the course of the vestibulocochlear nerve (adapted with permission from Grant, Basmajian (1965)).

e.g. the ear canal, ear drum, ossicle chain, or labyrinth windows. Sensorineural deafness is caused by any disease affecting the cochlea which turns sound energy into electrical signals, or the cochlear nerve which carries the signals to the brain. Some patients may have mixed deafness.

There are some clues to the cause of deafness from the history:

- Some patients with conductive hearing loss have paracusis, the ability to hear better in noisy rather than quiet surroundings. It is most typical of otosclerosis.
- Most people with sensorineural deafness complain that it is much harder to hear in a noisy environment and more intense sounds rapidly become unpleasantly loud, known as loudness recruitment.
- Sensorineural deafness is not helped by speaking more loudly. It particularly affects high frequencies.

Examination of hearing

Hearing by bone conduction measures the perceptive function of the eighth nerve and cochlea. If bone conduction is normal, hearing by air conduction shows the state of the conducting and amplifying system. Sound of the same intensity heard by air conduction is amplified and should be louder.

Whispered voice, or single words at arms length, made while making a masking noise in the other ear by rubbing the finger tips, will identify severe unilateral or bilateral deafness. This test is crude and poorly reproducible.

Tuning fork tests use a 256 or a 512 Hz fork. *Don't use a 128 Hz fork* because the note produced is too hard to distinguish from vibration.

Weber test

The fork is struck lightly to avoid overtones and its base placed on the forehead in the midline. If there is sensorineural deafness (e.g. there is a lesion affecting the perceptive mechanism), bone conduction is decreased on that side and the sound is heard loudest in the normal ear.

In conductive hearing loss, there is a lesion of the sound amplification mechanism and the sound is heard loudest and longest in the affected ear. One theory is that this is due to the effect of ambient noise "masking" the acuity of the normal ear.

Rinne test

The base plate of the ringing fork is placed on the mastoid until the sound is no longer heard and then the prongs of the fork are placed close to and in front of the ear canal. It should be heard for roughly twice as long by air conduction.

In normal people, air conduction, AC, is better heard than bone conduction, BC, owing to the amplification function of the tympanic membrane-ossicles. In sensorineural deafness, both are reduced, with AC is still better than BC because of the amplification produced by the intact conducting mechanism.

If air conduction is greater than bone conduction, then this is a "positive" Rinne result. In moderate or severe conductive hearing loss, bone conduction is greater than air conduction — a "negative" Rinne. False negative Rinne tests may occur in severe unilateral sensorineural hearing loss. The bone conduction may appear better than air conduction because the sound is conducted

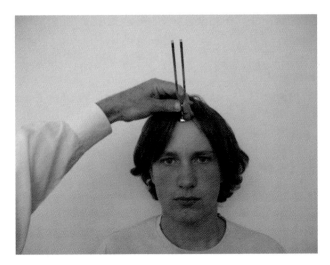

Figure 5.10.   Weber test.

from the mastoid through bone to the other ear. A "masking" sound in the other ear will help prevent this potentially misleading result.

Acoustic neuroma

Deafness is common and usually has no neurological significance. However, progressive unilateral sensorineural hearing loss and tinnitus are the most common presentation of an acoustic neuroma, an unusual benign tumour arising from the eighth nerve, but eventually compressing the brainstem and cerebellum. A pure tone audiogram will confirm sensorineural hearing loss and MRI scan is definitive. CT scan is not reliable in this condition.

Cranial Nerve VIII and the Vestibular System

The function of the vestibular system is to detect and signal motion and the effect of gravity in order to allow adjustments to posture and to maintain eye fixation on a particular point in space, despite small amplitude rapid movements of the head.

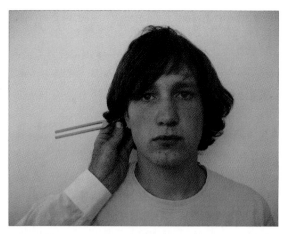

A

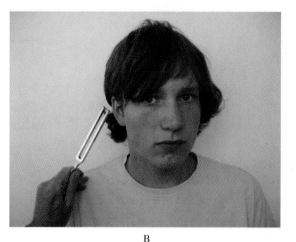

B

Figure 5.11. Rinne test. A: Testing bone conduction. B: Testing air conduction.

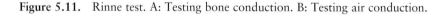

The three semicircular canals are at right angles to each other to detect head acceleration in any plane. The otolith organs detect the static effect of gravity and provide awareness of body or environmental tilt.

The vestibular sensors are connected via the vestibular nerve to the vestibular nuclei at the ponto-medullary junction and via them, have input to the spinal cord, cerebellum and to the centres for eye movement integration in the brainstem. Vestibular sensation is conveyed via the thalamus to the superior surface of the temporal lobe and the parieto-insula cortex.

The four most useful tests of vestibular function are: examination for peripheral vestibular nystagmus, the head-thrust test, heel-toe, "tandem", walking and the Dix–Hallpike manoeuvre.

Peripheral vestibular nystagmus

Peripheral vestibular nystagmus is fine, unidirectional, horizontal rotatory and beats toward the side opposite the lesion and is worse when looking to that side. It is inhibited by fixation and rapidly subsides over days to weeks, from central compensation for any permanent peripheral defect, but may still be detectable examining the fundus with fixation eliminated by closing the other eye. Hyperventilation and head shaking may also unmask peripheral vestibular nystagmus.

Head-thrust test

The head-thrust test reliably detects unilateral (or bilateral) horizontal semicircular canal hypofunction or failure. To test the right side, ask the patient to keep their eyes on your nose. Turn the head 20–30° to the left side and then rapidly turn the head towards the midline. A normal response is instant matched counter rotation of the eyes so that there is no detectable loss of fixation. In an abnormal response, the counter rotation of the eyes is either inadequate or absent, the eyes fail to remain on the target and move to the right with the head. The patient makes a visible fast voluntary eye movement to refixate the target. Similar tests can be done for the posterior and anterior canals, but are more demanding to perform, particularly in elderly patients with limited range of neck movement.

Heel-toe walking

People with acute unilateral vestibular lesions will often wander when heel-toe walking, typically, but not always, towards the side of the lesion.

The Dix–Hallpike manoeuvre

The Dix–Hallpike manoeuvre is a test for benign positional paroxysmal vertigo arising from debris in the posterior semicircular canal (PSC). The test is designed to activate the PSC by turning the head to the side so that the canal is in the plane of head movement, then vigorously stimulating the canal by moving the head through a 90° arc.

To perform the test, explain to the patient what you are about to do and that they should keep their eyes open and fixed on the bridge of the examiner's nose, no matter how dizzy they feel. Rarely the test may cause nausea and occasionally vomiting. Turn head to the side being tested. Move the patient quickly to a (slight) head hanging position.

In a positive test, nystagmus will occur after a short latent period of 1–5 seconds with its direction dependent on eye position. Looking towards the dependent ear, the nystagmus is predominantly rotational with the superior pole of the iris beating toward the affected ear. Looking ahead or to the opposite ear, the nystagmus is vertical, beating towards the top of the head. The duration of nystagmus is typically less than 30s (rarely it can be longer or even persistent, but these features suggest a central cause). Reversal of direction of rotation occurs on sitting up and nystagmus will fatigue (lesser duration of, or no nystagmus) on repeating the test. Benign positional vertigo can be treated effectively by immediately proceeding to an Epley manoeuvre.

Benign paroxysmal positioning vertigo: *Positioning* refers to the provocation of the symptoms by the sudden head movement, rather than the eventual head posture. The symptoms are due to a (dispersible) clump of debris in the PSC which causes prolonged stimulation of the cupula, briefly mis-signalling the brain. Debris adherent to the cupula is hypothesized to be a cause of positioning nystagmus which persists until the head position is shifted. Head vibration at the time of repositioning manoeuvres may be an effective treatment. BPPV arising from the PSC — the common form symptoms are most likely on lying down and especially on getting up, looking up or down, all movements most likely to stimulate the PSC.

Migraine is probably the most common cause of acute vertigo. Migraineurs have an increased frequency of vestibular events, thought still to be attributable to migraine. Vertigo may precede, occur with or be unrelated to acute migraine attacks. Symptom duration may vary from 30 minutes to several weeks and there may be no headache.

Acute peripheral vestibular lesion — vestibular neuritis. Incidence is 3/100,000/year. This is an idiopathic cranial mononeuropathy akin to Bell's palsy and to non-vascular sudden onset deafness. Although often proposed to be due to herpes simplex virus, a recent study of valacyclovir, methylprednisolone or both showed benefit only for methylprednisolone, suggesting an underlying inflammatory cause is most likely.

Meniere's disease

Incidence — 15/100,000 per year. The typical history is of tinnitus, which may be continuous, worse at the time of attack, often described as roaring like the sea or like listening to a sea shell. There is deafness and a sensation of fullness in the affected ear immediately preceding the acute attacks of vertigo. The vertigo is severe for minutes, and lasts several hours, with a feeling of dizziness or unsteadiness that may last several days. Nystagmus is horizonto-rotatory. The initial nystagmus beats toward then away from the affected ear, i.e. there is vestibular excitation followed by depression of function. The cause is thought to be increased volume of endolymph. Attacks may be due to rupture into perilymph. Gradual hearing loss develops in the affected ear, and a proportion develop bilateral disease. A key feature is fluctuation in low frequency hearing loss, the degree of impairment of vestibular function and tinnitus. Some patients develop drop attacks, called "Tumarkin" crises. Other causes of acute attacks of vertigo include vertebrobasilar territory transient ischaemic attacks and brainstem or cerebellar infarction. Cerebellar infarct or haemorrhage may present as severe vertigo and vomiting without brainstem symptoms. Infarct with occlusion of the internal auditory artery usually affects both hearing and vestibular function. AICA territory

infarction causes vertigo, vomiting, deafness, facial palsy and ipsilateral limb ataxia. The eye movement abnormalities are ipsilateral
gaze evoked nystagmus, impaired pursuit and vestibular nystagmus, reflecting infarction of the labyrinth, cochlea, vestibular nuclei
and vestibular cerebellum.

Vertigo is a common feature of brainstem lesions of multiple
sclerosis. There may be a history of previous typical episodes of
demyelination, or other central symptoms or signs. Nystagmus in
more than one direction or vertical nystagmus indicates a central
cause. A first episode of CNS demyelination affecting the eighth
nerve root entry zone may mimic an acute peripheral vestibular
lesion and is an unusual cause of isolated acute vertigo.

Bilateral peripheral vestibular disease/failure produces imbalance and oscillopsia. Oscillopsia is a sensation of the world moving on head movement due to an inadequate vestibulo-ocular
reflex. The patient complains of causing blurred vision not present
at rest and may describe vertical movement of the environment
when walking, together with unsteadiness walking in the dark, or
on uneven ground. The head thrust test of the horizontal VOR
test will demonstrate bilateral vestibular impairment. Visual acuity is normal at rest but very degraded with slow head oscillation.
When acute it is usually due to gentamycin toxicity, but may be
idiopathic.

Central causes of positional vertigo/nystagmus: Central nystagmus may be unidirectional and horizontal, but bidirectional or
vertical nystagmus is always central in origin. Positional testing
with head straight back over the end of bed, maintained for 60
seconds, may reveal downbeat nystagmus in a posterior fossa
lesion.

Common central vertigo

- Down beat nystagmus, provoked by head hanging, may occur
  with or without vertigo.
- Positional vertigo with purely torsional, or vertical nystagmus.
- Persistant positional nystagmus without vertigo.
- Positional vomiting without significant vertigo or nystagmus.

Head shaking nystagmus: Nystagmus occurring on shaking the head (with eye closed) may reveal vestibular asymmetry in a peripheral or a central lesion. Nystagmus induced by Valsalva may be caused by either a posterior fossa lesion or a communication between the middle and inner ear. A perilymph fistula due to round or oval window rupture may occur from loud noise, barotrauma, or Valsalva associated with exertion. A Valsalva raises middle ear air pressure via the Eustachian tube, causing symptoms because of the abnormal communication with the inner ear.

Chronic giddiness: A common cause is a decompensated peripheral vestibular lesion. When there is chronic dizziness and dislike of open spaces and crowds, with no signs on examination, the diagnosis is usually phobic vertigo.

Cranial Nerves IX and X: The Glossopharyngeal and Vagus Nerves

---

The examinable functions of the glossopharyngeal and vagus nerves are:

- Touch, pain and temperature from the pharynx, tonsils, soft palate and posterior 1/3 of the tongue.
- Taste from the posterior 1/3 of the tongue — seldom if ever tested in practice.
- Motor supply of the palate, pharynx and vocal cords.

Examination of cranial nerves IX and X

Listen to the voice. In soft palate weakness, it is nasal and there can be nasal regurgitation of fluid with nasal speech. With unilateral vocal cord paresis, it is soft and breathy.

Observe the soft palate movement on saying "Ah". Note that the uvula and soft palate often show minor asymmetry on movement in normal people.

Test the gag response by touching the posterior pharyngeal wall with a long cotton-tip (a microbiological swab is suitable). Observe the movement of the soft palate and the curtain movement of the posterior pharyngeal wall. Make sure you touch the posterior pharyngeal wall to test ninth/tenth nerve sensation when eliciting a gag response.

Ask the patient to cough. In normal larynx function, there is a brief explosive "huh" from forcing air through closed vocal cords. In vocal cord paresis, a prolonged softer bovine "herrr" is heard instead.

Other occasionally useful tests:

If speech is slurred, check articulation with "Pa, Ta, Ka". Labial, lingual and palatal aspects of articulation can be tested separately with phrases emphasising each: labial, "baby hippopotamus". Lingual, "West Register Street"; palatal, "lean, long and lanky".

Swallowing may sometimes be tested using tap water. Give a small test swallow using about 5 ml. Pay attention to any delay between the oral and pharyngeal phase. Listen for coughing in the 20–30 seconds after the swallow, and for a "wet" voice, both indicative of aspiration. If the test is successful with 5 ml, repeat the test with 30 ml of water.

Myasthenia is an important cause of difficulties with speech and swallowing. Reading a passage of text, or counting out loud may make fatigue of the jaw, tongue or palate obvious.

Direct inspection of the vocal cords

Most physicians do not have the equipment or skill to examine the vocal cords and although it is an important part of the evaluation of the vagus nerve, this will usually have to be arranged with an ENT service.

Cranial Nerve XI: The Accessory Nerve

Weakness of the sternomastoid on one side should be looked for when there are symptoms related to the lower cranial nerves. Bilateral weakness of neck flexion from weakness of both sternomastoids occurs with anterior horn cell disease, severe and usually inflammatory neuropathy, such as Guillain–Barre; myasthenia, myositis or myopathy, including myotonic dystrophy. Examining the 11th cranial nerve seldom provides useful additional information in routine examination.

Anatomy and physiology

The accessory nerve is pure motor and supplies the trapezius and the sternomastoid.

Look for a droop of the point of the shoulder, present in trapezius weakness. Check neck rotation and shoulder shrug. Ask the patient to rotate their head against pressure from the examiner's hand against the chin to check sternomastoid strength. The opposite sternomastoid will stand out and its strength can be assessed. Bilateral weakness causes weakness of head flexion and if severe, the head lags backward when attempting to sit up from lying supine.

Observe the symmetry of the shoulder girdle from the front and examine the position of the scapula and trapezius from behind. Look for a difference in the distance to the spinous processes and between the relative position of the upper and lower poles of the medial border of the scapula. Observe the bulk of the muscle at rest, during

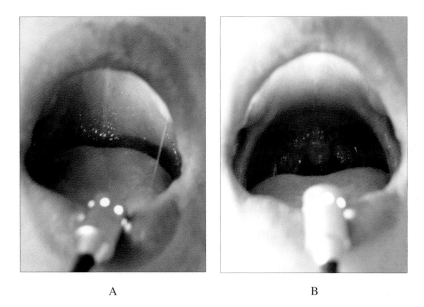

A   B

Figure 5.12.   Examining the palate. A: Palate relaxed. B: Palate on phonation.

shrugging — upper part; shoulder bracing — medial part; and on arm abduction (which may produce winging).

Herpes zoster with or without skin vesicles may affect any motor root or roots. The nerve may be affected as it passes through the skull base as part of the Jugular foramen syndrome. Surgical damage to the accessory nerve in the posterior triangle of the neck is usually obvious. The nerve supply to both muscles may be affected by acute brachial neuritis which is probably the most common idiopathic cause. This syndrome causes severe pain in the neck and arm for days to a few weeks followed on recovery by recognition of weakness in affected muscles. Unilateral weakness of these muscles may pass unnoticed and be discovered later during fitness or weight training.

Cranial Nerve XII: The Hypoglossal Nerve

The hypoglossal nerve contains only motor fibres to the tongue muscles. At least half the pyramidal tract fibres are crossed. Unilateral tongue lesions may cause difficulty moving food around in the mouth and a tendency to bite the weak side. Bilateral lesions cause difficulty with rapid clear speech and with swallowing, presumably by interfering with bolus propulsion into the pharynx.

Careful examination is especially important when there is a history of bulbar difficulties (with swallowing and speech) and for fasciculation where motor neuron disease is a possible cause of limb weakness without sensory loss.

Examining the hypoglossal nerve

Listen to speech and inspect the tongue — relaxed in the floor of the mouth for wasting or fasiculation, on protrusion for deviation. The tongue is responsible for clarity of the "Ta" sound in "Pa Ta Ka", a rapid effective test of articulation.

In unilateral LMN lesions, on protrusion the tongue deviates toward the weak side from the unopposed effect of the contralateral genioglossus and atrophy produces deep longitudinal folds in the mucosa. Weakness can be confirmed by testing the ability to

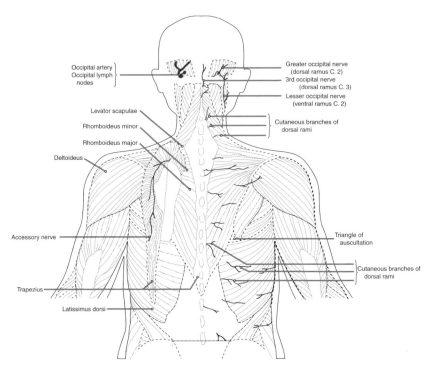

Occipital artery
Occipital lymph
nodes

Greater occipital nerve
(dorsal ramus C. 2)
3rd occipital nerve
(dorsal ramus C. 3)
Lesser occipital nerve
(ventral ramus C. 2)

Levator scapulae

Rhomboideus minor

Rhomboideus major

Deltoideus

Cutaneous branches of
dorsal rami

Accessory nerve

Triangle of
auscultation

Cutaneous branches of
dorsal rami

Trapezius

Latissimus dorsi

A

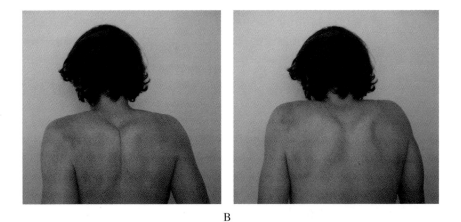

B

Figure 5.13.   Examining trapezius. A: Its anatomy. B: Shoulder Shrug.

pushing the tongue into the cheek and exert pressure against the examiner's finger. Flaccidity and wasting can be confirmed by palpation.

Fasciculation may be present and is only reliable when observed with the tongue relaxed in the floor of the mouth. Tremulous fasciculation-like movement may be seen in normal people on contraction and many find it difficult to relax the tongue for long. It is often best not to draw attention to the tongue and care is necessary before concluding fasciculation is present.

Myasthenia gravis is an uncommon but important cause of bilateral tongue weakness that is easy to misdiagnose. Myasthenic tongue weakness can be detected by having the patient count aloud. Tongue function may be affected rarely by tumour or amyloid infiltration.

A unilateral lesion of the pyramidal tract between the lower pre-central sulcus and the hypoglossal nucleus in the medulla can produce unilateral tongue weakness and dysarthria that is usually transient. A common cause is the dysarthria/clumsy hand syndrome seen in lacunar infarction in the posterior internal capsule.

Bilateral upper motor neuron tongue weakness causes marked slowing of tongue movements and characteristic spastic speech which is slow and effortful. The tongue looks small and tight and moves poorly and slowly either on repeating "la la la" or on rapid side-to-side movement. Any bilateral lesion of the pyramidal tract may be responsible. Motor neurone disease is a common cause.

Further Reading

Danesh-Meyer HV, Savino P, Sergott R. The correlation of phenylephrine 1% with hydroxyamphetamine 1% in Horner's syndrome. *Br J Ophthalmol* 2004; 88: 592–593.

Grant J, Basmajian JV. *Grant's Method of Anatomy* 1965; 7th edn. The Williams & Wilkins Company: Baltimore.

Gray H. *Anatomy of the Human Body* 1918; Lea & Febiger: Philadelphia.

Hodges JR. *Cognitive Assessment for Clinicians* 2007; 2nd edn. Oxford University Press: Oxford.

156   D. Abernethy

Homans J. *A Textbook of Surgery* 1940; Springfield Illinois.
Leigh RJ, Zee DS. *The Neurology of Eye Movements* 2006; 4th edn. Oxford University Press: New York.
Miller NR, Newman NJ, Biousse V, Kerrison JB. *Walsh and Hoyt's Clinical Neuro-Ophthalmology: The Essentials* 2008; 2nd edn. Lippincott Williams and Wilkins: Baltimore.
The Guarantors of Brain. *Aids to the Examination of the Peripheral Nervous System* 2005; Elsevier Saunders: London.

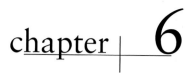

chapter 6

The Nervous System: Part II

David Abernethy

Examination of the Peripheries

The neurological examination of the peripheries, is usually performed, and recorded, in the order:

- Power
- Tone
- Reflexes
- Sensation
- Coordination

As with all examinations, much can be made by watching the patient as they enter the room, observing them as they give a history and observing from the end of the bed before the commencement of the formal examination.

Kichu's thoughts . . .

Greet the patient outside the room and walk behind them. It will give you invaluable information.

Inspection

Each muscle should be inspected and/or palpated during power testing. If the person has weakness as the diagnostic problem all clothing except underwear should be removed.

Look carefully at the weak muscles and compare sides when the other is unaffected. Commonly wasted muscles include: the small hand muscles (1DIO and APB), quads, calves and anterior tibial muscles (note prominence of the anterior tibial border when they are wasted). When neuropathy is suspected, examine the small muscles of the hand and foot (abductor hallucis and extensor digitorum brevis) in particular, as wasting is common there.

CASE STUDY 6.1

A 57-year-old man is noticed by his wife to have reduced movement of his right arm and leg for up to two years. For at least six months, he notices some difficulty brushing his teeth and with buttons.

The clinician thinks "The arm and leg both involved so the lesion is likely in the cervical spine, brainstem or brain (Where). The onset can't be dated, closer than the last 1–2 years. There was no acute incident at the start and he has got slowly worse — what was initially only apparent to his wife has begun to be noticeable to him."

"…The answer to 'What is the lesion?' is that it's a gradual process affecting the motor pathway — therefore it could be a neurodegenerative process or a tumour — but there is no headache, seizures or mental dulling." On examination, he is generally slow moving, with reduced spontaneous movements and the right foot seems to flop slightly. The right arm does not swing when walking. He has reduced piano playing finger movements, fatigue of amplitude and breakdown of rhythm of alternating pronation and supination in his right hand. There is no right arm or leg weakness, or reflex asymmetry. There is no tremor but he has cogwheel rigidity in his right arm.

Further examination demonstrates extrapyramidal slowness, fatigue of repetitive movements and rigidity confirming the suspicion of typically unilateral onset idiopathic Parkinson's disease without tremor as the cause of the problem. It refutes the possibility of a hemiparesis by failure to find weakness, reflex change or extensor plantar response in the right limbs. There is also no focal weakness to account for the slight drop foot walking. The importance of the mode of onset and progression to accurate clinical diagnosis is emphasised.

Watch for fasciculation in relaxed muscles. Calf fasciculation is common in apparently normal older people. In primary muscle disease, facial weakness and a hyperlordotoic posture may be useful clues.

Gait

It is good practice to greet the patient in the waiting area and introduce yourself. Politely insist on carrying their bag, coat, magazine etc. to free their arms and walk behind them to the consulting room. This brief social interaction provides useful insight into mental status and personality, as well an ideal opportunity to assess akinesia, bradykinesia, ataxia, gait and rest tremor with the patient relaxed and in as natural a state as possible. When reasonable, the same applies to inpatients. The insight gained is invaluable in rapidly orienting the doctor to the likely cause of the problem.

There are a number of easily recognized gait disturbances:

Lower motor neuron foot drop: There is increased lift of the knee, so the drooped foot clears the ground and the foot slaps down.

Stamping: From loss of posterior column function (rare and usually due to neuropathy, previously to meningovascular syphilis)

Hemiparesis: The arm may be carried partially or fully flexed and the leg is stiff, circumducted slowly and the toes catch the floor.

Spastic: Due to hereditary spastic paraplegia. The knees are adducted, the feet intorted and plantar flexed and dragged forward stiffly and slowly. In other forms of bilateral leg spasticity, the changes are similar, but less severe.

CASE STUDY 6.2

A 70-year-old obese man has had weakness in his legs worsening over four months. He has been barely able to walk with a frame for a month. His feet feel numb and hot. He has urinary urgency that has

> *(Continued)*
> worsened over the last month. There is no back pain. He is referred for nerve conduction studies.
>
> The clinician thinks "Numb, hot feet with leg weakness could be a neuropathy and he is obese, which might mean he has diabetes mellitus as the underlying cause. The duration is compatible with a relatively severe neuropathy." (Where and What). "... If he can't walk because of neuropathy, his hands should be weak too and his leg reflexes should be absent and plantars down or unresponsive." (a possible inconsistency in the Where hypothesis). "...Urinary urgency in the elderly is common, but might indicate a spinal cord problem." (an alternative 'Where' hypothesis). On examination cranial nerves, arms and hands are normal. He has severe leg weakness for hip flexion, extension and knee flexion. Tone in the legs is spastic, the reflexes are brisk, plantars extensor and pinprick is perceived as blunt on feet and legs to T6/7 on the anterior chest wall.
>
> Examination shows the weakness is upper motor neuron type, and clearly discriminates between a peripheral neuropathy and a spinal cord lesion, indicating the latter.

Ataxia: The gait is wide based, unsteady turning and the patient cannot walk heel to toe.

Spastic ataxic gait: The gait is wide based and there is slowness and evident spasticity on one or both sides. This is most common in secondary progressive multiple sclerosis.

Early Parkinson's disease: The affected arm does not swing and tremor may be evident. The shoulder on the affected side is high. The leg is over flexed at the hip and there may be a subtle tendency for the foot to slap, resembling foot drop of lower motor neuron type.

Advanced Parkinson's disease: The arms are held stiffly at the sides, the body is flexed, steps are small and the base is narrow. Turning requires multiple movements.

Limb girdle muscular dystrophy: There is a hyperlordotoic posture and waddling due to hip abductor weakness, causing the pelvis to drop when the leg on that side is taken off the floor to take a step. When severe, the person needs to perform Gower's manoeuvre to get up from the floor or a bench — pushing their body up with their hands on their legs and thighs.

Apraxia of gait: Also known as *Marche à petits pas* (walking with small steps). The base is broad, and on starting there is a phenomenon referred to as gait ignition failure, in which the person jiggles from one foot to the other as if the feet are stuck to the floor, before taking an effective step. Walking proceeds with short, wide-based steps.

Tone

It takes some practice and experience to appreciate the tone disturbances seen in upper motor neuron, lower motor neuron and extrapyramidal syndromes. Identifying tone disturbances is extremely valuable and may be the single most useful clinical observation in a patient with conditions such as foot drop or bilateral leg weakness.

There are five useful types of tone disturbance:

- Hypotonia in LMN lesions.
- Spasticity in UMN lesions.
- Extrapyramidal rigidity.
- Cog wheeling without rigidity seen in moderate or severe action tremor.
- Motor negativism or Gegenhalten, seen particularly in encephalopathy, in dementia, and to a mild degree in otherwise apparently healthy elderly.

The issue is most often whether there is increased or decreased tone due to an upper or lower motorneuron lesion. For this purpose, tone in the arm should be tested by pronating and supinating the wrist, at the same time unpredictably flexing and extending the arm vigorously at the elbow. In spasticity, there is a "catch" on supination of the forearm and on extension at the elbow. When severe, this catch is likened to the initial difficulty then less force needed to open the blade of a pocket knife. Rolling the leg from side to side will demonstrate spasticity, rigidity or hypotonia at the ankle. Rapid flexion at the knee will bring out a spastic catch.

Abrupt dorsiflexion of the ankle *while the knee is flexed* is the most sensitive way to detect ankle clonus. A few beats of clonus may be seen in normal persons with brisk reflexes. Sustained ankle clonus is probably always abnormal.

When an extrapyramdial disorder is suspected, either because of bradykinesia or tremor, a different technique, with slow flexion and extension of the fingers, wrists and pronation and supination at the elbow is more sensitive. The rigidity can be enhanced by simultaneous voluntary up and down movement of the abducted contralateral arm. Plastic resistance to movement that doesn't change in intensity during movement, likened to bending a lead pipe, is typical in Parkinson's disease. There are often a superimposed series of ratchet like jerks known as "cog wheel" rigidity.

Action tremors also produce cog wheeling but without rigidity. This causes most difficulty in moderate or severe essential tremor, drug induced tremor and particularly in unilateral dystonic hand tremor with ipsilateral arm bradykinesia. Lack of fatigue of alternating fingers to thumb apposition movement can be useful to distinguish Parkinson tremor from this condition.

Testing the Power of Muscles

The principles of power testing

Instructions should be short, simply worded, supplemented by a visual demonstration of the required movement.

Test power across just one joint so that just one muscle or functional group is being tested at a time. This means, for example, when testing biceps, grip the lower forearm, not the hand. If the wrist is weak, attempts to test biceps will fail.

Kichu's thoughts . . .

Testing the motor power is made easy by explaining in simple terms and then demonstrating to the patient. This will save time and create less confusion.

Support and stabilise the limb proximal to the joint across which the movement is being tested, particularly if it is weak. For example, when testing finger extension, support the palm with your left hand while pushing down over the proximal PIP joints with your right.

Work from shoulder to fingers and hip to toes to remain organised. In general, you test flexion and extension at each joint, except the shoulder. For speed and efficiency, test both/all movements at one joint in one limb, then compare the same movements in the other. When weakness is extensive, it can be helpful to write down the results as you go before you forget, using the MRC scale, and then moving on to the next joint.

Any muscle is most powerful when fully contracted and should be tested in this position except for elbow and knee extension, when the joint should be tested slightly flexed by 30–40 degrees to avoid locking. In the recommended positions, the normal muscle is usually stronger than an examiner using reasonable force.

The key decision the examiner must make for each movement or muscle tested is whether it is normal or weak. Failure to make this distinction with confidence both movement-by-movement, while also paying attention to the distribution of weakness, is a common serious deficiency in examinations and in clinical practice. Casual reports that "limb strength is 4/5" frustrates analysis of the likely causes of the weakness by comparison with the expected pattern of muscle or joint movement weakness that discriminates between lesions of pyramidal tract, root, plexus component, peripheral nerve, neuromuscular junction or muscle.

The MRC scale:

- Full power   5
- Weak   4
- Movement against gravity   3
- Movement with gravity eliminated   2
- Flicker   1
- None   0

The MRC scale is most useful for monitoring the progress of an illness. The degree of weakness is typically not the point; it is the distribution and significance that matters. The most serious progressive paralyzing illnesses begin with slight weakness.

Examining Muscle Groups

The exact technique of examining the different muscle groups and the "patter" by which the patient is instructed are equally important to contract the muscles being tested.

Shoulder abduction

Instruction to person being examined: "Put your arm up like this — *demonstrate* — keep your arm up, don't let me push it down."

Examiner's action: Push downward on the elbow, i.e. on the distal arm, to get maximum leverage. You should not be able to overcome the muscle with reasonable force.

Elbow flexion

Instruction: "Bend your arm up like this. Pull your fist towards your nose. Don't let me straighten it."

Examiner's action: Allow the person to almost fully flex the arm (not well shown in the illustration). Support the elbow with one hand (this is important in weak patients) and attempt to straighten the

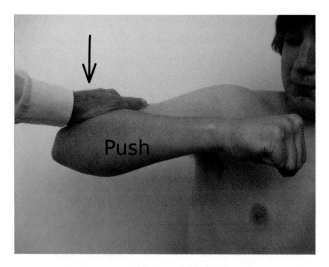

Figure 6.1.   Deltoid C5, C6 axillary nerve.

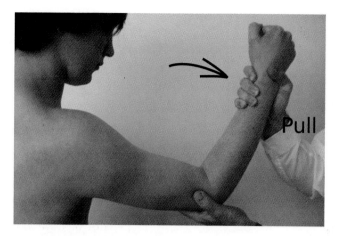

Figure 6.2. Biceps C5, C6 musculocutaneous nerve.

flexed, supinated forearm, pulling on the lower forearm, *not* the hand. The forearm should be supinated to decrease the effect of brachioradialis.

Elbow extension

Instruction: "Push (your arm) to me. Don't let me bend it."

Examiner's action: Support the arm at the elbow and holding the forearm at the wrist, push toward them. Allow them to extend their arm beyond 90 degrees or it may appear weak. Alternatively, to demonstrate subtle weakness, have the person hold their elbows in to their sides with forearms flexed at 90 degrees. Holding both wrists, pull upward as they push down. Weakness of one or both sides will be obvious.

Wrist extension

Instruction: "Keep your wrist back (like this), don't let me pull it down/straight."

Examiner's actions: Hold the lower forearm with one hand and firmly attempt to straighten the dorsiflexed wrist with the other.

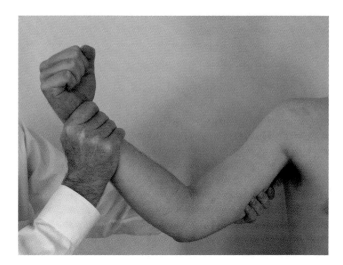

Figure 6.3.   Triceps C6, C7, C8 radial nerve.

Wrist flexion

Instruction: "Keep your wrist down (like this), don't let me pull it up/straight."

Examiner's actions: Hold the lower forearm and firmly attempt to straighten the flexed wrist with your other hand. Wrist flexion is not a critical part of screening arm strength. Disproportionate weakness of wrist and finger flexion is a striking feature of the chronic condition inclusion body myositis, often encountered in specialist clinical examinations.

Finger extension

Instruction: "Keep your fingers out straight, don't let me bend them."

Examiner's actions: This is a test of extension at the MCP joints. It is important to support the palm and apply pressure over the PIP joints *not more distally*, because extension at the PIP and DIP joints is performed by the small hand muscles.

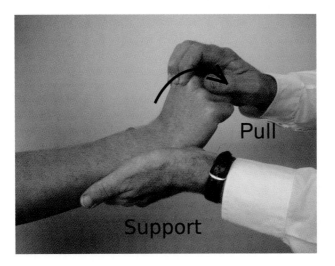

Figure 6.4. Extensor carpi radialis C5, C6 radial nerve extensor carpi ulnaris C7, C8 posterior interosseous branch, radial nerve.

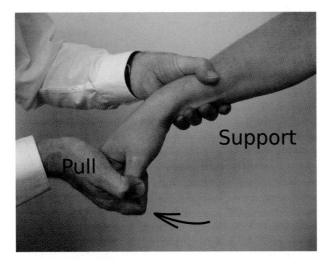

Figure 6.5. Flexor carpi radialis C6, C7 median nerve. Flexor carpi ulnaris C7, C8, T1 ulnar nerve.

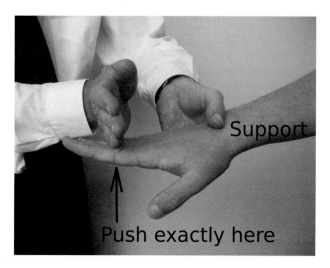

Figure 6.6. Extensor digitorium C7, C8 posterior interosseous branch, radial nerve.

Finger flexion

Instruction: "Curl your fingers like this and don't let me straighten them."

Examiner's actions: Attempt to straighten the flexed fingers. Having the patient grip two of the examiner's fingers is an inferior technique. Flexion occurs at the MCP, PIP and DIP joints performed by the intrinsic muscles of the hand, the flexor digitorium superficialis and the flexor digitorium profundus, respectively.

Testing flexion of the individual distal phalanges is particularly informative in ulnar neuropathy. If fingers 4 and 5 are involved, the lesion is likely localised to the elbow. Isolated weakness of flexion of the distal phalanges of fingers 1 and 2 implies a lesion of the anterior interosseous branch of the median nerve, most often due to brachial neuritis.

Finger abduction

Instruction: "Spread your fingers apart (like this), push your index finger towards your other hand. Don't let me push it back."

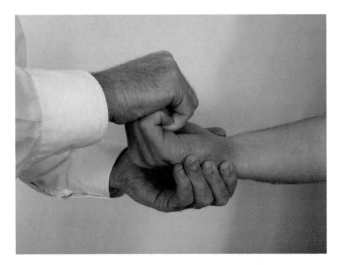

Figure 6.7. Flexor digitorium superficialis C7, C8, T1; median nerve. Flexor digitorium profundus Cu, C8 F2, three median nerves, F4, five ulnar nerves.

Examiner's actions: Push on the index finger at PIP joint level towards the other fingers. Hold the other fingers with your other hand. Almost all people are able to resist reasonable force applied to the index finger at this point, but will give way if force is applied further distally. Look at the first dorsal interosseous muscle and palpate it with your other hand. It is usually only necessary to test the first dorsal interosseous muscle to establish whether the ulnar nerve function is intact and for Horner's syndrome, 1DIO and APB, with a check for sensory loss on the medial forearm to assess T1 integrity.

Thumb abduction

Instruction: "Hold your hand out like this, push your thumb towards your other hand/leg, don't let me push your thumb down on to your hand."

Examiner's actions: Push down on the thumb over the IP joint. Look at and palpate the muscle. The intention is to test Abductor Pollicis Brevis to assess median nerve function. The thumb must be abducted in a plane perpendicular to the palm to eliminate the influence of abductor pollicis longus as much as possible.

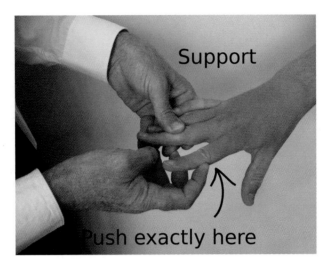

Figure 6.8.   First dorsal interosseous C8, T1 ulnar nerve.

Hip flexion

Instruction: "Lift your leg up like this, don't let me push it down."

Examiner's actions: Push towards the foot. This movement is often poorly performed, particularly by older women, so that detection of weakness may not be reliable. When obviously weak, the person will be seen to lift their legs onto the bed using their hands.

Hip extension

Instruction: "Keep your leg on the bed. Don't let me lift it."

Examiner's actions: Pull up under the heel, and if needed knee. The patient's buttocks should be lifted off the bed if they are fully exerting themselves. Effort, even with vigorous exhortation is often inadequate. In hysterical weakness of one leg, inadequate effort during voluntary hip extension can be demonstrated by checking for an increase in downward heel pressure when the opposite hip is flexed against resistance (Hoover's sign — inconsistency between hip extension tested directly and indirectly).

Knee extension

Instruction: "Push your leg out straight."

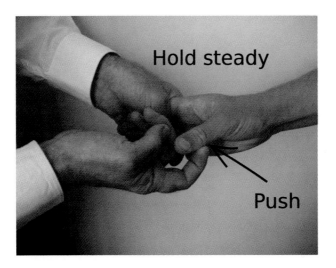

Figure 6.9.   Abductor pollicis brevis C8, T1 median nerve.

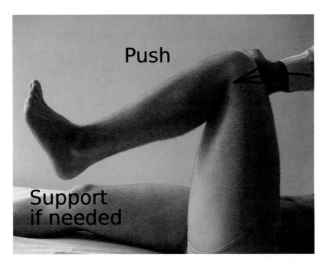

Figure 6.10.   Iliopsoas L1, L2, L3 spinal nerves and femoral nerve.

Examiner's instructions: Allow the knee to be slightly flexed, at 135–150 degrees, and try to bend it more as the patient attempts to straighten it. Make sure the foot is not catching on the bed. If done with the leg straight, the knee will lock, preventing testing of Quadriceps power. Be careful of the skin around the ankle which

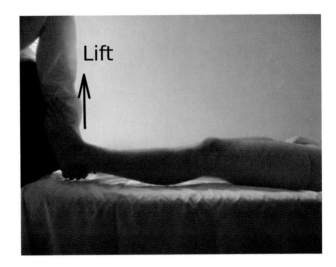

Figure 6.11.   Gluteus maximus L5, S1, S2 inferior gluteal branch or sciatic nerve.

may be fragile and the shin tender in older people. Very vigorous testing can cause fracture.

Knee flexion

Instruction: "Bend your leg and don't let me straighten it."

Examiner's instructions: Support the knee with one hand and attempt to straighten the flexed leg with the other hand holding the ankle. Often poorly performed.

Ankle inversion

Instruction: "Twist your foot inwards, (like this) and don't let me straighten it."

Examiner's actions: Inversion and eversion are often difficult movements to explain to the patient. Attempt to overcome the inversion and twist the foot from inverted to a dorsiflexed position.

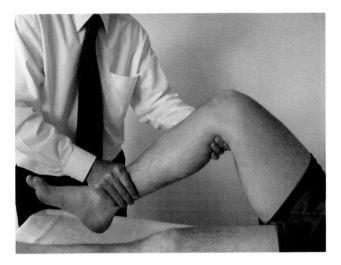

Figure 6.12.   Quadriceps femoris L2, L3, L4 femoral nerve.

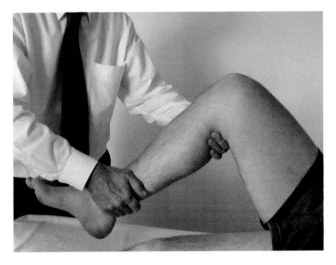

Figure 6.13.   Hamstrings L5, S1, S2 sciatic nerve.

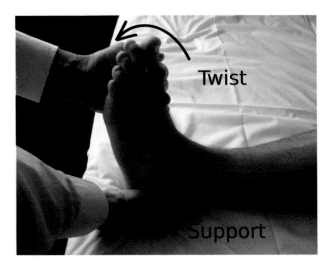

Figure 6.14.   Tibialis posterior L4, L5 tibial nerve.

Ankle dorsiflexion

Instruction: "Keep your leg on the bed and pull your toes up towards your head."

Examiner's actions: Push very firmly along the line of the leg against the distal metatarsals in an effort to overcome the movement. This a strong muscle and the leverage should be the maximum possible as you watch the person's face to ensure the test is not painful.

Ankle eversion

Instruction: "Twist your foot outwards, don't let me straighten it."

Examiner's actions: Attempt to overcome the eversion of the foot, with pressure applied to the MTP region.

Ankle plantar flexion

Instruction: "Push your foot down, don't let me push it up."

Examiner's actions: This is a powerful muscle and the examiner should exert enough force to move them bodily on the couch. The

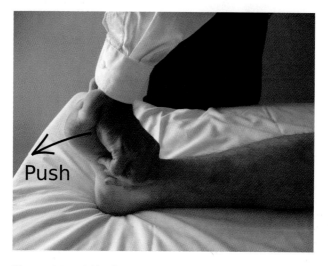

Figure 6.15. Tibialis anterior L4, L5 deep peroneal nerve.

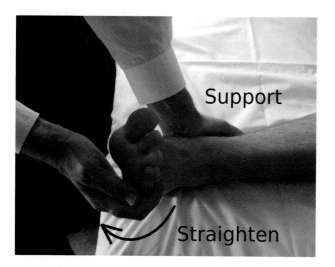

Figure 6.16. Peronei L5, S1 superficial peroneal nerve.

most effective test is to have the patient attempt to stand on tip toe of the leg under test while the other foot is off the ground. At the same time, look for wasting of the posterior calf muscles. In persons with functional weakness of foot plantar flexion on bedside testing,

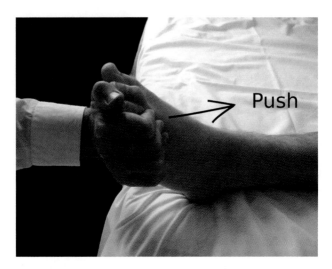

Figure 6.17.   Gastrocnemius S1, S2 tibial nerve.

the ability to walk on tiptoes provides unequivocal evidence of inadequate effort during the examination.

In plexopathies and nerve injuries, it may be useful and necessary to examine a greater range of muscles. Diagrams of the plexi, nerves and muscles can be found in the monographs "Aids to the examination of the peripheral nervous system" and "Nerves and nerve injuries".

Aids to the examination of the peripheral nervous system, nerves and nerve injuries.

Patterns of Muscle Weakness

Hemiparesis

A pyramidal tract lesion weakens the muscles that allow the decorticate posture to develop, with adducted shoulder, flexed forearm, wrist and adducted, flexed fingers. The leg is an adducted, rigid pillar with a plantar flexed, inverted foot. Even subtle pyramidal tract damage causes particular loss of ability to make rapid, fine finger to thumb and toe tapping movements that are a useful screen in the rapid assessment of ill patients.

Paraparesis

Bilateral leg weakness due to pyramidal tract lesions with sensory loss and bladder disturbance is usually due to a spinal cord lesion. Recognition is critically important since failure to diagnose and treat spinal cord compression promptly has severe consequences.

Peripheral nerve injuries

Peripheral nerve injuries, compressions and radiculopathies are common in practice and have well-defined distributions of weakness and sensory loss.

Nerve root lesions typically have pain in the spine radiating down a sclerotome into a limb, the trunk and, less frequently, the neck or head. There is usually tingling, numbness and often sensory loss inside the area-affected dermatome. Weakness affects muscles innervated by that myotome, but varies in severity and is often subtle due to overlap in innervation of individual muscles by several myotomes. There will be reflex depression only if there is a reflex affected by the damaged root.

Focal peripheral nerve lesions cause weakness of innervated muscles and sensory loss confined to their described territories. Focal lesions may be painful, with pain at any site along the nerve, typically radiating into the sensory distribution of the nerve if touched or tapped at this point (Tinel's sign).

Axonal sensorimotor peripheral neuropathy

This form of peripheral neuropathy, when, as typical, length dependent, causes stocking and then glove-pattern of sensory loss. Weakness of dorsiflexion of the feet typically precedes weakness of the small muscles of the hands with both median and ulnar innervated muscles equally affected.

Demyelinating peripheral neuropathy

Weakness is typically both proximal and distal in demyelinating neuropathy often referred to for this reason and because of radicular back pain and raised CSF protein as a polyradiculoneuropathy.

Plexopathies

Idiopathic brachial and lumbosacral plexopathies are typically accompanied by severe pain at onset, with weakness of individual proximal muscles outside the territory of any one nerve root or peripheral nerve. Weakness is often not noted until the pain improves, occasionally not until months later.

Muscle disease

In myopathies, a proximal pattern of weakness is most common with weakness of neck flexion, shoulder abduction, hip flexion and difficulty performing a "sit-up", or a rise from a squat. Some muscle diseases have more specific patterns; for example, in inclusion body myositis, finger flexors and knee extensors are often particularly severely affected. It pays to think about and record the strength of individual movements mainly for careful pattern analysis as an aid to diagnosis and also as a record for future comparison.

Common Causes of Weakness in the Limbs

Ulnar nerve

Ulnar neuropathy from compression at the elbow produces weakness of abduction of the fingers but not the thumb, weakness also of the long flexors to the 4th and 5th fingers. There is often wasting of the interossei and sensory loss on the ulnar border of the hand, stopping at the wrist, splitting the fourth finger. Weakness of the adductor pollicis can be demonstrated with Froment's sign — when AP is weak, flexion of the distal phalanx of the thumb is required to grip a card between the adducted thumb and index finger.

Median nerve

Median nerve compression in the carpal tunnel results (when severe) in weakness and wasting of abductor pollicis brevis, with numbness affecting the palmar surface of fingers 1, 2, 3, and lateral 4. Sensory symptoms are usually more marked at the finger tips. In mild cases, tingling and pain develops in the hand, spreading up the arm with use of the hand and the person is woken with similar symptoms at night, relieved by hanging the hand down.

Common peroneal nerve

A common peroneal nerve lesion, when due to compression at the fibula head, is painless, usually sudden and marked foot drop, weakness of dorsiflexion and eversion with normal inversion (provided by tibialis posterior innervated by L4 and L5) and numbness on the lateral leg and dorsum of the foot. Sensory loss is usually subtle. Ankle jerk is normal.

To separate an L5 root lesion from a peroneal nerve palsy, look at internal rotation of the hip, performed by Gluteus Medius, L4 and L5 and at foot inversion, L4 and L5; as for dorsiflexion, but inversion is mainly performed by the tibialis posterior muscle innervated by the tibial nerve. Dorsiflexion is mainly done by tibialis anterior, supplied by the peroneal nerve. In peroneal nerve palsy, internal rotation and ankle inversioin are normal.

Reflexes

Deep tendon reflexes test the local reflex arc and when the reflex arc is intact, the state of upper motor neuron inhibition can also be assessed. Examination is a critical part of localisation of weakness, nerve and root lesions (see previous sections). In peripheral neuropathies, loss of reflexes is thought to reflect involvement of the large amplitude sensory fibres. In purely motor peripheral nerve diseases, reflexes tend to be preserved until there is extensive muscle loss.

Superficial (abdominal) reflexes disappear in upper motor neuron lesions.

It is important that the muscle be relaxed when obtaining the reflex. It is usually easiest to do the test with the person lying on a couch. When the reflex appears absent, reinforcement manoeuvres can enhance the reflex. Clenching the teeth can be used for the arms and pulling one hand against the other in a "sailor's" grip for the legs. If the person holds their ankle rigid, contracting tibialis anterior, the tendon can be seen and felt. A useful trick to obtain relaxation of the ankle dorsiflexor and some facilitation is to ask the person to push down lightly with the ball of the foot.

Reflex	Segment(s) tested
Biceps, supinator	C5–6
Triceps	C7
Finger flexor	C8
Knee jerk	L3–L4
Ankle jerk	S1

Biceps reflex

With the arm relaxed, flexed to 90–120 degrees, Place your thumb on the biceps tendon and strike your thumb with the hammer. If possible for the left biceps, reach over the person, place your *left* thumb on the biceps tendon.

In very large people, lift the arm up on to the chest, supporting it at the elbow with your left hand while keeping your left thumb on the tendon.

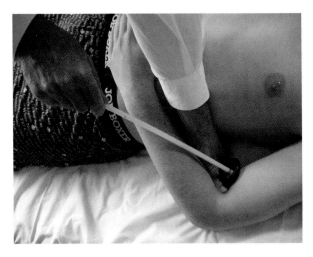

Figure 6.18.   Left biceps reflex.

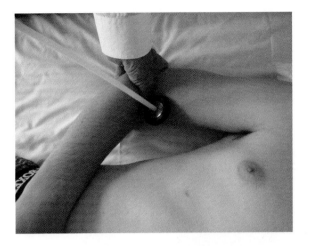

Figure 6.19.   Right biceps reflex.

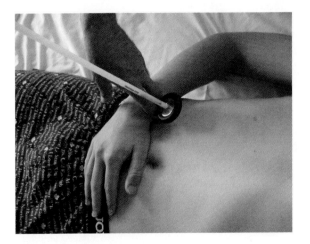

Figure 6.20.   Right supinator reflex.

Supinator reflex

Place two fingers on the distal radius and tap them with the hammer. Look for contraction in brachioradialis.

In patients with very brisk reflexes, there may *also* be flexion of the fingers and thumb. This is often, but not always, pathological, i.e. evidence of an upper motor neuron lesion. In an inverted supinator reflex, there is no brachioradialis contraction, but the hyperexcitable cord below leads to finger flexion. This implies both a local cord lesion and a C6 radiculopathy, most often due to cervical spondylosis.

Triceps reflex

Make sure the arm relaxes against the chest, then tap the tendon 3–5 cm above the olecranon. Look for contraction in the triceps muscle.

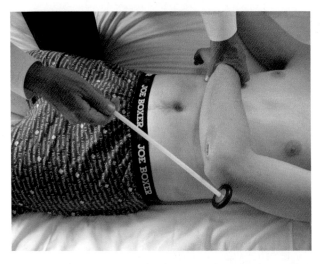

Figure 6.21.   Left triceps reflex.

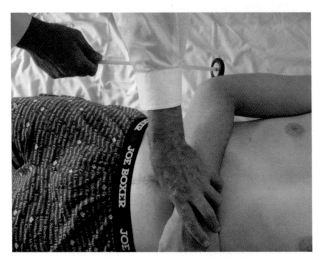

Figure 6.22.   Right triceps reflex.

Finger flexor reflex

Ask the patient to flex their fingers lighty. Apply gentle tension and tap on your fingers. The fingers should contract, although the response may be minimal in normal people.

Knee jerk

The legs should be relaxed and flexed at least 30 degrees. Tap the tendon between the patella and tibial tuberosity.

Look for contraction of the quadriceps.

Ankle jerk

Flex and abduct the hip, passively flex the ankle to at least 90 degrees, more in young people. Watch that tibialis anterior is not contracted (see above). Tap on the Achilles tendon 3 cm above the calcaneus. This is usually the most useful reflex and it is worth going into some trouble to learn to examine it reliably.

Plantars

Start gently with a pointed but not sharp object, such as a rounded-off tip of a tendon hammer, pen or key. Increase intensity if

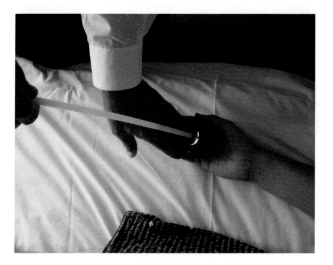

Figure 6.23. Finger flexor reflex.

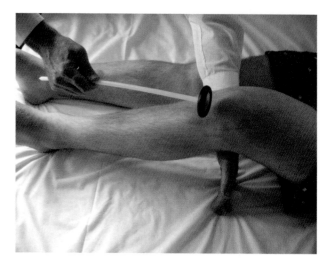

Figure 6.24.   Left knee reflex.

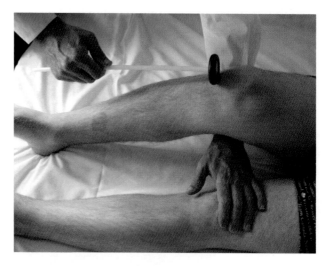

Figure 6.25.   Right knee reflex.

needed. Scratch up the lateral sole and across the ball of the foot. Be gentle, start softly. You can always do it harder a second time if needed.

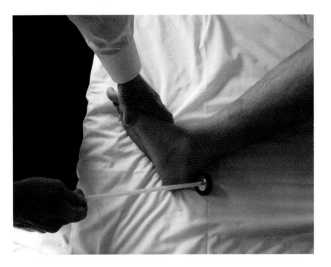

Figure 6.26.   Right ankle reflex.

Superficial abdominal reflexes

These reflexes are not very important. Remember these disappear in a pyramidal tract lesion and are mainly used in an attempt to demonstrate subtle spinal cord involvement above L3 and below C8. A cord lesion above L3 will cause brisk knee and ankle jerks. If it is higher than C8, the finger jerks will also be brisk. There are no tendon breaks between these two levels. Lightly stroke along the line of the abdominal dermatomes towards the midline on each side with a cotton tip or pen. The local external oblique muscle should contract. These are not present reliably in the obese, the elderly or the multi-parous.

Radial nerve

A common radial nerve injury is known as "Saturday night palsy". The patient is often young, has been intoxicated and wakes unable to dorsiflex the wrist, or extend fingers or thumb. Abduction of fingers often appears weak. As a result of diffuse hand weakness not obviously due to a single nerve and onset during sleep, acute stroke is often suspected. The apparent weakness outside the radial nerve territory disappears when finger abduction is tested with the forearm and hand laid on a flat surface to provide passive finger extension.

T1 root lesions and combined lesions of median and ulnar nerve

In combined lesions of both median and ulnar nerve, weakness is in the same distribution as for T1 root lesions, but with sensory loss in the median and ulnar territories of the hand, rather than the medial border of the arm and forearm. Such lesions are much more common than a T1 root lesion. Horner's syndrome may occur with proximal lesions of the T1 root.

Cervical radiculopathies

C6 radiculopathy weakens elbow flexion and wrist extension. Sensory symptoms and loss is on the dorsolateral forearm, thumb and index finger.

C7 radiculopathy gives pain from neck, shoulder arm and forearm, weakness of elbow, wrist and finger extension, with sensory symptoms and numbness that may be localised by the patient in the middle three fingers. To distinguish a C7 root lesion from a radial nerve palsy, look at pronation. The median nerve innervates pronator teres but the segmental innervation comes from the C6 and C7 roots.

Radiculopathies and nerve lesions affecting the lower limb

S1 radiculopathy causes pain in the low back, lateral buttock, thigh, leg, and foot; numbness on the lateral border of the foot, with weakness (usually mild) of gluteus maximus, hamstrings, plantar flexion and eversion of the foot, with numbness on the lateral border and depressed or absent ankle jerk. Weakness is best demonstrated by asking the person to lift their bodyweight onto tiptoe (with the other foot off the ground). The examiner may need to help them retain balance.

L5 radiculopathy causes pain in the low back, lateral buttock, thigh, leg, and foot, numbness on the medial border of the foot involving the big toe, with weakness (usually mild) of glutei, hamstrings, inversion and dorsiflexion of the foot. The ankle jerk is not affected.

Sensation

Sensory testing is of most value when one of the conditions or problems discussed in more detail below is suspected either from the history, or from findings during the examination. Suggested effective approaches to sensory examination are given for each common scenario. Don't waste time on sensory testing. Anticipate that the information may be confusing and not particularly reliable. Do the tests once, carefully and adapt to any resulting uncertainty by incorporating it explicitly into your formulation. Sensory testing is very subject to suggestion and unconscious cues from the examiner. Techniques that try to avoid this are described below. In particular, it is worth asking the patient to report the sensation they feel in response to a stimulus, rather than to leading question such as "Is this sharp? Vibrating?" etc.

When the issue is a screening examination in a patient where sensation is expected to be normal, test position and vibration of fingers, then toes, that cotton wool can be detected with eyes closed and pinprick is reported sharp after a single adequate stimulus to the three divisions of the fifth nerve, the distal dorsum of fingers 1, 3 and 5 and toes 1 and 5. These are more than adequate to exclude most neuropathies, both large and small fibre; radiculopathies, spinal cord lesions and disassociated and chequerboard patterns of sensory loss. Each test can be completed in a few seconds.

Joint position sense and vibration

The tests are straightforward, so get them done first and quickly. Structuring the tests in the order and manner suggested can speed up the process by reducing misunderstandings while avoiding the need for lengthy explanations. Test perception of position at the PIP joint of the index finger first on each hand. This is seldom abnormal and the movement is easier for the patient to perceive. It has the effect of familiarising them with the test before moving on to the usually more important test of perception at the great toes.

Technique for joint position sense

During position sense testing, hold the digit being tested by the sides to avoid giving pressure cues. Explain "I'm going to move your finger up and down. This is up, this is down. Close your eyes. I want you to tell me in *which direction* I move your finger. *Towards* up or *towards* down" (makes the response "middle" less likely). Make one non-confusing large movement, then progressively smaller single movements for each test. Wait for their response after each movement, but avoid cueing their responses — i.e. just wait, resist the temptation to ask for a response. Make the direction of these movements unpredictable. Do the same for the big toes.

In persons who either cannot or will not relax or who respond "up ... down ... up ... down" no matter what movement of the toe, abandon the test, perform a Romberg test of dorsal column function as a screen and consider the issue in light of their overall problem, sensory tests, reflexes, walking and balance.

The performance of elderly patients on this test is so poor, it is frequently a waste of time. If position sense is impaired in the fingers, move to the wrists and elbows. If absent in the toes, test at ankle and knee. Patients who deny position sense in their limbs, but have normal reflexes and no apparent defect of limb use, balance or walking, are quite frequently encountered in whom the problem is not due to nervous system disease. Patients with no perception of position sense in the fingers should have pseudoathetosis (writhing movements of the fingers) holding

> **Kichu's thoughts . . .**
>
> Sensory examination is tiring for the patient and the doctor. Ask the patient about the symptoms and have a hypothesis before you start the testing. It is said that the best neurologist is the one who knows which sensory sign to ignore.

arms outstretched with eyes closed. When JPS is absent in the toes and definitely absent at the ankles, performance on the Romberg test should be affected.

Technique for vibration sense

As for JPS, vibration sense is more easily perceived in the fingers, where it is much less often affected. Test distally first, at the index finger DIP joint. As with all sensory testing, it is occasionally more informative to ask the patient firstly "What do you feel?" Expect "vibration, humming" or similar, but anticipate "cold or pressure" when the patient cannot perceive vibration. If not felt at the DIP joint, test the other side before testing more proximally. This circumvents the occasional essentially normal patient who reports to feel nothing to one knee, then reports vibration from the other MTP joint. Test in the upper limbs successively until felt, beginning with the DIP joint of the index finger, moving proximally to the MCP joint, wrist, lateral of epicondyle humerus and lateral clavicle. In the legs, test until felt by the patient successively at the MTP joint, the medial malleolus, anterior tibial tuberosity, the anterior superior iliac spine and then each rib in turn from T10. There is no need to test proximally once the patient has confidently reported feeling vibration distally. In elderly patients, vibration sense is not uncommonly absent in the legs and pelvis without obvious explanation. Both a neuropathy and a spinal lesion could theoretically be responsible. Often neither are apparent.

Light touch and pin prick

Test from the insensitive to normal skin. It is easier for the patient to recognise the distinction. If the affected area is hypersensitive, test from the normal to the hypersensitive area. Pin prick is often the most useful modality to test. It is a good idea to ask the patient to report what they feel. You may get a surprise. "I don't feel pricking, it is just like something pushing" or it may be hypersensitive. Temperature sensation is not usually tested.

Reported numb areas

Ask the patient to outline any area of numbness. This is often enough to make the diagnosis on its own and often provides the most reliable information about the boundaries of an area of sensory alteration. The patient's report of the area of sensory loss is likely to be more precise than your examination. Get the patient to map out the loss, moving from insensitive to normal feeling. Make sure they demonstrate the relevant discriminating boundaries between peripheral nerve or dermatome territories without suggestion from you if possible.

Then test with the eyes closed. Test from reduced sensation to normal. Don't try to draw a complete map. The issue is to distinguish the possible causes suggested by the history and other findings such as the motor weakness. Test at the relevant boundaries to separate the diagnostic options for the sensory defect reported or discovered on examination. This depends on the clinical problem, but is often a simple issue such as distinguishing L5 from S1 in a patient with back pain and a numb foot, L5 from peroneal in a patient with foot drop and numb anterolateral leg and medial foot; the first and third divisions of the trigeminal nerve, V3, from C2 in a patient with facial numbness that may be due to a trigeminal nerve lesion.

Sensory Syndromes

For dermatomal or peripheral nerve sensory loss, the area the patient reports affected must be compatible with a known nerve territory and not cross into adjacent nerve territories — this is what you should be aiming to determine by examination. For example, for the ulnar nerve, the sensory loss should end at the wrist and split the fourth finger. More extensive loss, including the third finger and extending more than a few centimetres up the medial forearm, suggests a C8 root lesion.

You only need to know the accepted boundaries of the median, ulnar, radial, peroneal, tibial and lateral cutaneous nerve of thigh for a good working knowledge. In more unusual lesions, refer to the diagrams by Haymaker and Woodhall (Haymaker *et al.*, 1953).

Because of the overlap of adjacent dermatomes, the area of demonstrable sensory loss is often much less than expected from dermatome charts in radicular lesions. The periphery is usually more affected than the strip from spine down the limb. When possible aim tests to cross from the numb area to potentially normal at pre- or post-axial lines where there is a transition between widely separated dermatomes, and the distinction from abnormal to normal may be abrupt.

There are only a few spinal roots that are frequently affected — C6, C7 and C8 in the arms and L5 and S1 in the leg. Pain in the spine, radiating down the limb is a frequent and highly suggestive accompaniment.

Peripheral neuropathy (axonal, length dependent)

The patient is often not aware of sensory loss. Vibration sense is usually affected, position is sometimes affected. When testing light touch and pin prick, begin distally with eyes closed. Ask the patient at the outset of testing (but not during it) to report each time the cotton wool touches the skin and after they detect each pin prick, including if it is sharp. Expect a stocking, glove pattern.

Spinal cord lesions

Detection of a sensory level is critical to clinical diagnosis and choice of site for imaging. The patient may not be as aware of the sensory loss, which is usually not total, although awareness is quite variable.

Begin on the foot with a pin. Ask the patient to report what he feels, which if abnormal, is likely to be touching, rather than pricking. Move consistently up the body, gently pricking once every 2–3 cm or so, asking for report of sensation changing or becoming normal. Keep going until a level is discovered or excluded. After testing the front of the lower limb, then trunk, move at the C4/T2 boundary to the inner arm, down the medial arm and forearm, across the distal dorsums of the fingers and thumb, then up the lateral arm to the neck, posterior scalp, over the ear on to the face, then across the cheek to the nose. Then look for sacral sparing, seen in intramedullary lesions, by working up the back of the legs to the perianal area.

Sensory loss in stroke syndromes

The sensory loss pattern is seldom very critical to diagnosis except for thalamic and lateral medullary lesions. Both produce interesting patterns. Sensory loss of central origin is often more apparent on hand, foot and face than trunk.

Dissociated sensory loss occurs in syringomyelia, lateral medullary syndrome and Brown–Sequard hemi-spinal cord lesion. Light touch, JPS and vibration sense are unaffected, but pin prick and temperature are absent in the affected areas.

Coordination

The effects of cerebellar disease depend on the location of the lesions and their speed of onset. The lateral lobes control the smooth movement of the limbs. The inferior cerebellum controls eye movements. Damage to the superior paravermal areas affect speech. Pathological processes confined to the midline or vermis typically affect walking and the stability of the trunk when sitting and have little or no effect on limb coordination. When cerebellar disease is severe, particularly when paraneoplastic, the patient may not be able to stand or sit. Cerebellar disease may produce tremor most obvious when attempting accurate placement of the finger or heel on a target. Tremor can affect the head at rest, referred to as titubation.

Examination for cerebellar disease includes listening to the patient talk, watching them walk, noting any truncal instability during arm power testing and testing limb coordination. Hearing is relevant to a number of causes of ataxia. The corneal response is relevant if a cerebellopontine lesion is suspected.

Speech, when affected, has a telegraphic quality. When severely affected, repeating "Pa, Ta, Ka" (labial, lingual and palatal consonants) degrades to "baa daa gaa" (Posner, 1995).

Gait

When there is mild truncal ataxia, walking heel to toe for 10 steps may bring out the impairment. This test is often not performed well by older patients and is frequently abnormal in functional illness and must be interpreted with caution in light of the overall problem. Similar comments apply to the Romberg test. When more severe, gait is broad based and may be particularly unsteady turning.

Romberg test

Ask the patient to stand with feet together and eyes closed. It pays to stand with arms encircling the patient, ready to catch them, should they begin to topple. It is intended to detect unsteadiness due to position sense loss, but can also be abnormal in cerebellar disease, or in an acute vestibular lesion.

Tests of limb coordination

Finger-nose-finger test

The patient should touch the examiner's finger, then their nose, then finger again. If the ataxia is severe, the patient should touch their shoulder to avoid striking their face. There may be tremor accentuated

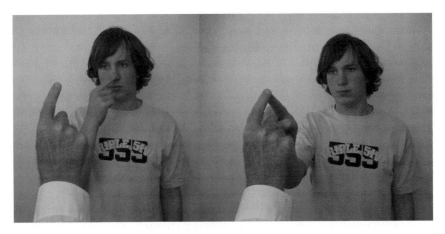

Figure 6.27. Finger-nose-finger test.

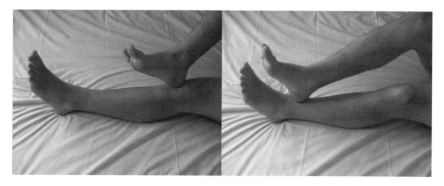

Figure 6.28.   Heel-shin test.

as the target is approached and clumsiness during the whole of the movement.

Heel-shin test

It is important the patient be asked to lift the leg high and then to place the heel precisely on the anterior tibial tuberosity (or any defined point on the leg) to accentuate any intention tremor as the heel approaches the knee; then run smoothly and quickly but not carelessly down the anterior tibia.

Dysdiadokinesis tests

Tapping the back of one hand alternately with the palmar and then dorsal surfaces of the fingertips of the other is the most commonly used test. Other similar tests include: small amplitude rapid tapping of the fingertips of one hand on the dorsum of other hand and making small regular circular polishing movements of the fingertips of one hand on the dorsum of other hand. The rhythm and amplitude is typically erratic.

Eye movements in cerebellar disease

Eye movement abnormalities can provide unequivocal evidence that the cerebellum is involved in the ataxia. Testing may show hypometria, hypermetria, broken pursuit and gaze-evoked nystagmus, both in horizontal and vertical gaze. Anticonvulsant toxicity is the most commonly encountered cause. Lesions in the region of the foramen magnum may produce downbeat nystagmus. This is typically worse looking to the side and down. When subtle, it may be evident only during ophthalmoscopy. Downbeat nystagmus is idiopathic in about 40%, due to cerebellar degenerations 20% and to Arnold Chiari malformation in 7% (Wagner *et al.*, 2008).

Cerebellar causes of ataxia

- **Acute causes**
  - Stroke, multiple sclerosis, Wernicke's encephalopathy

- **Subacute causes**
  - Parneoplastic — rapid onset over days to weeks and progression to severe disability
  - Cerebellopontine angle tumours (see eighth nerve section)
  - Cerebellar tumours

- **Chronic causes**
  - Hypothyroidism
  - Multiple system atrophy
  - Cerebellar degenerations
  - Spino cerebellar degenerations, i.e. Fredriech's ataxia with absent reflexes, extensor plantars and loss of position sense

- **Unusual or rare chronic causes**
  - Metabolic disease such as cholestanolosis, with deposits in the Achilles tendon
  - With deafness, mitochondrial disease, Refsum's (deafness, ataxia, demyelinating peripheral neuropathy, ataxia, ichthyosis), Haemosiderosis from subtle insidious bleeding into the subarachnoid space from a cavernoma, AVM or unknown cause

Non-cerebellar causes of ataxia

Acute peripheral vestibular lesions can cause severe unsteadiness, but the overall circumstances and particularly the horizontal vestibulo-ocular reflex, or head thrust test, aid in distinguishing the conditions. Inferior cerebellar infarction is an important differential diagnosis of acute vertigo when the HVOR is normal.

Any cause of severe position sense loss can cause ataxia as the most apparent defect, seen in sensory variants of Guillain–Barre, subacute combined degeneration secondary to vitamin B12 deficiency which frequently presents as a subacute or acute onset sensory ataxia and in dorsal root ganglionitis, most often associated with connective tissue disease, particularly Sjogren's syndrome. When position sense loss in the arms is severe, the person may have writhing finger movements with arms held out, fingers extended and eyes closed (pseudoathetosis).

Spinal cord compressive lesions occasionally present with gait ataxia as the apparent problem.

Movement Disorders

Hypokinetic movement disorders cause akinetic rigid syndromes or parkinsonism. The key features are:

Akinesia, a reduction in spontaneous movements, slowness or bradykinesia, rigidity, an involuntary increase in tone, affecting both agonist and antagonist muscles (e.g. the flexors and extensors, or the pronators and supinators of the wrist). The tone increase is plastic and may have a cogwheel element, particularly when there is tremor.

Hyperkinetic movement disorders have increased movements either spontaneously, as a result of voluntary movement or after a stimulus. Most are involuntary, but tics, akathisia (motor restlessness associated with antipsychotic drugs) and restless legs may be partly voluntary.

Types of hyperkinetic movements

Tremor: A sinusoidal oscillation of a body part as a result of alternating or synchronous contraction of agonist and antagonist muscles.

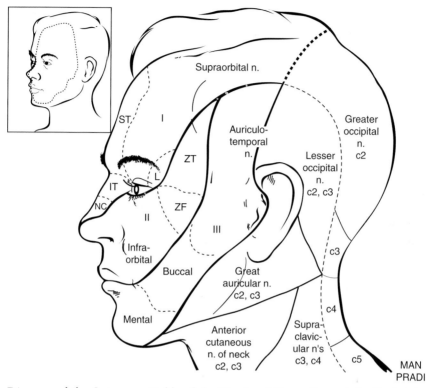

Diagram of the Cutaneous Fields of the Head and Upper Part of the Neck. The fields supplied by the three divisions of the trigeminal nerve (I, ophthalmic; II, maxillary; III, mandibular) are indicated by heavy lines, and their respective subdivisions by light broken lines. The conjunctivae are innervated by the ophthalmic division. Abbreviations refer to the following nerves: *B*, buccal; *IT*, infratrochlear; *L*, lacrimal; *NC*, external nasal branch of the nasociliary; *ST*, supratrochlear; *ZF*, zygomaticofacial; *ZT*, zygomaticotemporal. The lateral and superior boundaries of the posterior primary rami are indicated by broken lines.

Figure 6.29. Peripheral nerves of head and neck (adapted from Gray (1918)).

Myoclonus: Sudden shock like jerks, typically from muscle activation. Myoclonus can occur spontaneously at rest, be provoked by action, or be reflex in response to sensory stimuli. It can arise at spinal, brainstem, subcortical or cortical level. Myoclonus is most commonly seen in encephalopathy from drugs or sepsis and as a feature of epilepsy, parkinsonism or dementia. Asterixis, usually due

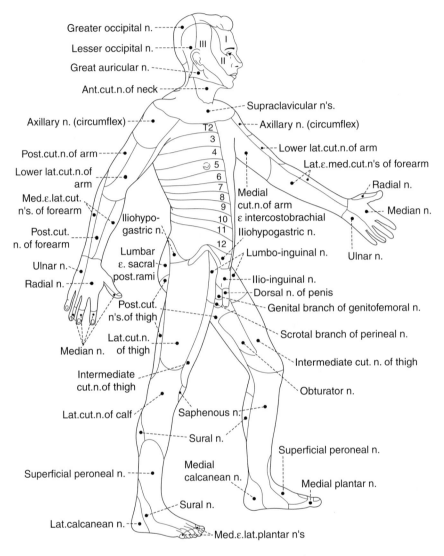

Figure 6.30.   Peripheral nerves lateral view.

to CO_2, drug or hepatic encephalopathy, is a form of myoclonus due to sudden inhibition of muscle tone.

Dystonia: An involuntary sustained muscle contraction, often co-contraction of agonist and antagonist, producing writhing twisting

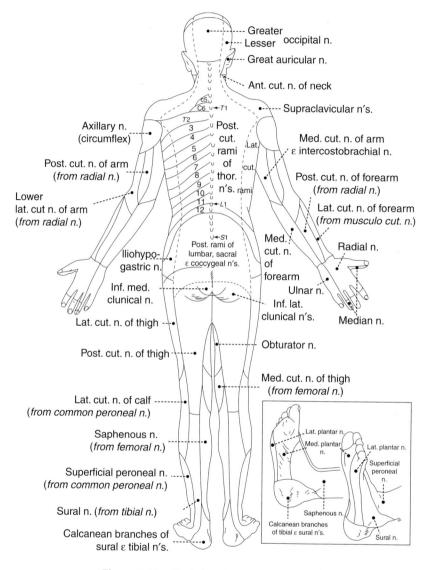

Figure 6.31. Peripheral nerves posterior view.

repetitive movements, abnormal sustained postures and at times, jerking. Dystonia can be provoked by action, and at times paradoxically relieved by voluntary movement or by a sensory trick. In cervical dystonia, placing a finger lightly against the chin can relieve

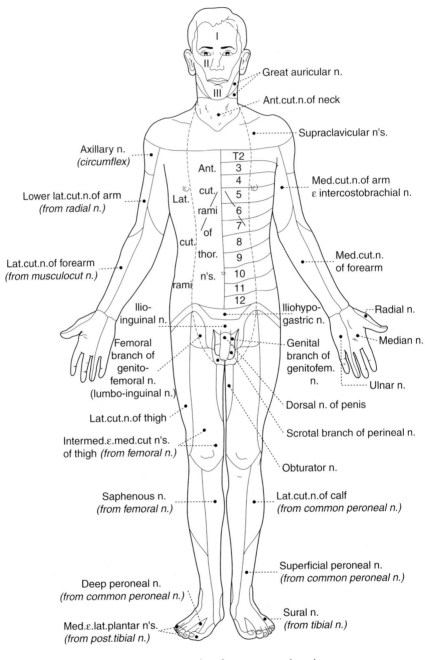

Figure 6.32.   Peripheral nerves anterior view.

the persistent twisting of the head to one side. Dystonia is most often seen as a feature of Parkinson's or after stroke or other focal brain lesions. It may be genetic, and occurs in an extensive list of rare genetic, metabolic and mitochondrial disorders.

Chorea: Involuntary small movements of the distal limbs and face that flit randomly from one part to another, and often incorporated into gestures by the patient to disguise the movement. Generalised chorea is most commonly encountered in the lupus anticoagulant syndrome, Huntington's disease and, rarely, in Sydenham's chorea.

Ballismus: Is a more severe form of chorea with violent flinging movements of the proximal limbs. It is usually unilateral, beginning acutely after infarction of the subthalamic nucleus.

Tics: Repetitive, stereotyped movements or vocalisations that can be briefly suppressed voluntarily. Patients often experience an inner urge, relieved by performing the tic. On the other hand, they persist during sleep.

Parkinsonism

Patients with Parkinson's disease have a characteristic lack of spontaneous and expressive movement, evident when sitting and in conversation, with reduced gestures, head and neck movement, blinking or eye movements. Their voice is soft and expressionless.

Rest tremor may be obvious in the waiting room, typically affecting one hand and the ipsilateral leg. Watching the patient walk to the examination area can be very helpful. In early Parkinson's disease, the limb involvement is usually asymmetrical, the hand tremor often appears while they are walking and the arm on the affected side does not swing as well, or at all. In slightly more advanced PD, the leg will be affected walking, usually being lifted higher at the hip, somewhat resembling the gait of a person with footdrop. In more severe PD, with bilateral involvement, getting up from the chair may take several attempts and an additional push up with their arms. When walking, the posture is flexed and step size reduced. Gait remains narrow based, even when balance is affected.

Bradykinesia can be demonstrated by making large amplitude, repetitive flexion movements of all fingers against the thumb, piano playing finger movements, or hand pronation supination movements on the thigh. The fluency of repetitive movements deteriorates and the amplitude declines distinctively with repeated movements, referred to as fatigue.

Severely affected patients have impaired postural reflexes. Test postural reflexes by giving a sharp pull backwards, whilst standing behind the person prepared and ready to prevent them falling down. A normal response is up to two small steps to maintain stance. The typical abnormality is either multiple small steps continuing backwards until stopped by the examiner, i.e. festination backwards, or a slow topple without reflex correction, with a fall inevitable unless prevented by the examiner.

Mood, mental status, eye movements and autonomic control of blood pressure on standing are all commonly affected in Parkinson's disease and related syndromes.

Tremor

Tremor is categorised by the situation in which it is most obvious: rest, posture or during movement. Some tremors are present in more than one situation.

Rest tremor is evident with the limb relaxed and completely supported against gravity.

- **Action tremors**
  A. Postural with the limbs outstretched
  B. Kinetic evident during the finger-nose test
  Terminal tremor is seen at the end of movement, present in most action tremors.

Intention tremor increasing in amplitude throughout movement as the target is approached, typical of cerebellar disease.

Tremors are sometimes called dystonic or myoclonic tremor because of the underlying condition rather than the clinical tremor type. Dystonic tremor in the hands tends to be asymmetric, jerky and worse in particular hand positions.this can be detected by slowly pronating and supinating the outstretched arms.

There are also task specific, position specific and isometric tremors. Writing tremor is the most common task specific tremor.

- **Rest tremor**
  Rest tremor is typically due to Parkinson's and is present in about 70% of cases. The leg on that side is usually affected. Tremor may often be seen in the hand while walking. The tremor usually disappears on performing an action such as maintaining a posture with the hands outstretched. When severe, Parkinsonian tremor may reappear this position after a brief lag of a few seconds, a so-called "emergent tremor". Marked action tremor may still be seen at apparent rest unless the limbs are at complete rest, fully supported and relaxed, either lying with hands resting on the lower abdomen or sitting with them resting in the patient's lap. Both rest and action tremor can be brought out by a mental task — such as saying the months of the year backwards with eyes closed.

- **Action tremor**
  The most common form of action tremor is enhanced physiological tremor, accentuated by stress or by drugs such as adrenergic agents, Lithium, valproate, steroids, drug or alcohol withdrawal, rarely by hyperthyroidism, and very rarely by hypoglycemia or pheochromocytoma. Tremor is not evident at complete rest (see caution above) and visible with hands outstretched, hands slightly dorsiflexed, fingers slightly separated. It may be slightly more apparent with the hands held near the mouth, when drinking from a cup and during the finger-nose-finger test.

- **Essential tremor**
  Prevalence estimates are highly variable from 3 to 40/1000, possibly as high as 14% over age 65, reflecting difficulty distinguishing physiological tremors. Typically, it does not affect legs. About

50% have a family history, and it may be improved by alcohol. It is similar to physiological tremor, but with age, the tremor increases in amplitude and slows in frequency. Tremor may affect head and voice as well as hands. Test for voice involvement by asking the patient to sing a sustained note (e.g. "EEEEE") and listen for an obvious rhythmic quaver. Action tremor can be identified and quantified by having the person write and trace a spiral with both hands.

Striking accentuation as the finger approaches the target is typical of a cerebellar tremor which is not usually evident at rest or on maintaining a posture. Cerebellar disease may also produce a regular head tremor (titubation).

Demyelinating neuropathy is an important but unusual cause of an action tremor. The patient may or may not be weak, the reflexes are usually absent.

Autonomic Function

Autonomic function is often affected in Parkinson's and in neuropathies, particularly in diabetes and amyloidosis. Orthostatic hypotension, defined as a systolic blood pressure (BP) reduction of at least 30 mmHg within three minutes of standing, is a key feature.

Autonomic failure can cause headache, with prolonged standing leading to blackout. It can be readily identified with simple equipment, using a test battery published by Ewing (Ewing *et al.*, 1982).

Further Reading

Edwards M, Quinn N, Bhatia K. Parkinson's disease and other movement disorders. *Oxford Specialist Handbooks in Neurology* 2008; Oxford University Press: Oxford.

Ewing DJ, Clarke BF. Diagnosis and management of diabetic autonomic neuropathy. *BMJ* 1982; 285: 916–918.

Graham J, Martin M (Eds.). *Ballantyne's Deafness* 2001; 6th edn. Whurr Publishers: London.

Gray H. *Anatomy of the Human Body* 1918; Lea & Febiger: Philadelphia.

Haymaker W, Woodhall B. Peripheral nerve injuries. *Principles of Diagnosis* 1953; 2nd edn. WB Saunders Company: Philadelphia.

Posner JB. *Neurologic Complications of Cancer* 1995; FA Davis: Philadelphia Co. 111.

Posner JB, Saper CB, Schiff ND, Plum F. 2007 *Plum and Posner's Diagnosis of Stupor and Coma*. Oxford University Press: USA.

Wagner JN, Glaser M, Brandt T, Strupp M. Downbeat nystagmus: Aetiology and comorbidity in 117 patients. *J Neurol Neurosurg Psychiatry* 2008; 79: 672–777.

chapter 7

Rheumatology

John Van der Kallen

Introduction

Musculoskeletal problems can be a localised problem to this system itself, or it can be signs of a systemic disease. History is invaluable in helping to differentiate this. Patients often present with pain. It is important to take a proper history of the pain — its character, duration, location, severity, whether it fluctuates and the exacerbating and relieving factors. It is important to decide if the pain is musculoskeletal, neurological or referred.

The history should particularly identify if there has been trauma and if so, the mechanism of the trauma. For instance, trauma to an ankle could be a direct blow resulting in a fracture or an inversion injury resulting in a ligament tear. Both can be equally painful!

The distribution of the joints involved is important.

> **Kichu's thoughts . . .**
>
> An acutely swollen and hot joint is infection until proven otherwise. Aspiration of the joint is needed.

If the pattern involves first carpometacarpal joints and hips, then one would think of osteoarthritis. However, if the metacarpophalangeal joints and wrists are involved, then one thinks of rheumatoid arthritis.

The chronicity of the complaint and any preceeding illness might also give clues. If a complaint began overnight, then one will think of infection or gout rather than the onset of rheumatoid arthritis.

Associated features such as fever, weight loss, dry eyes or mouth (sicca complex), skin rashes, fatigue, sleep disturbance, miscarriages, swollen lymph glands, headache or swallowing difficulties are also helpful. Finally, we need to know if there are other organs involved outside the musculoskeletal system. Therefore, quick screening questions regarding the respiratory, cardiovascular, gastrointestinal and neurological systems are needed.

The history will help the examiner decide which part of the examination is most important. In most situations with diffuse joint symptoms, nearly all the joints will need to be examined. It would be difficult to do extensive examinations of each joint in most clinical situations. Therefore, a quick examination will identify problematic joints. These joints can then be examined in more detail. Of course, if the patient comes with symptoms in only one joint, then it is usually sufficient to examine the joint. However, beware of systemic illness presenting as a single joint problem! A good example of this is psoriatic arthritis presenting as recurrent Achilles tendonitis.

Essentials of a Rheumatological History

- Which joints are involved?
- How long has the patient had the problem?
- Are the symptoms inflammatory or mechanical in nature?
- Was there a preceding illness or injury?
- Are there associated features?

The musculoskeletal examination requires careful observation. It requires a good knowledge of the anatomy and locomotor function. The signs can often be quite subtle. For instance, the range of movement maybe reduced in only one particular joint. Unless the joints are systematically examined, the decreased range of movement may remain undetected. Similarly, signs of inflammation can be missed unless each joint is carefully examined.

A rheumatological diagnosis or differential diagnosis can be made with a good history and examination. The diagnosis can be confirmed with subsequent investigations.

How to Reach a Rheumatological Diagnosis

- History
- Examination
- Investigations (usually X-rays and serology)

This chapter will describe the musculoskeletal examination of a number of joints and how to put them into clinical context so that a rheumatological diagnosis can be made.

CASE STUDY 7.1

A 78-year-old woman presents with two months of pain and stiffness in her hands. She has had intermittent pain in the past; however, these recent symptoms are persistent. She finds it is particularly difficult in the morning. She has difficulty making a cup of tea because her hands "won't work". She has taken some diclofenac which helps for a few hours. On examination, you notice that it is hard to see her metacarpophalangeal joints because of the swelling.

How would you come to a diagnosis in this patient? What are the important pieces of information that you need?

Hand Pain

A careful history is invaluable in diagnosis. Of course, this is not always possible in an exam situation. It is important to define where the patient has the hand pain. Is it in the wrists or is it in the fingers? Is it in the joints or soft tissues? Similarly, the character of the pain is important. Nerve compression syndromes often give a burning or shooting quality to the pain whereas arthritis usually gives an aching feeling with warmth and stiffness to the joints.

The duration of symptoms is important. Many rheumatological problems develop over a period of months and often, years. However, there are rheumatological problems that can develop overnight, such as gout or infection.

As with other joint problems, it is important to know if other joints are involved rather than just the joint or joints that the patient complains about. A careful history will often unveil a more diffuse problem than was previously suspected. The pattern of this joint involvement will often point to a diagnosis. For instance, 90% of patients with rheumatoid arthritis will have synovitis that affects the metacarpophalangeal (MCP) or wrist joints in a symmetrical pattern.

After taking the history, the clinician should have formulated a differential diagnosis.

The clinical examination helps to differentiate between these diagnoses. To begin the examination of the hands and wrists, the patient must be properly positioned. The hands and wrists must be exposed to at least the elbow. Placing a patient's hands on a pillow is ideal.

Common Causes of Wrist, Thumb and Finger Pain

Wrist

- Hypermobility
- Inflammatory arthritis (synovitis)
- Tenosynovitis (e.g. De Quervain's tenosynovitis)
- Osteoarthritis
- Fracture
- Bone lesions (malignancy, infection, avascular necrosis — mostly scaphoid)

Thumb

- Osteoarthritis (especially carpometacarpal and scapho–trapezium joint)
- Skier's thumb (tear of ulnar ligament of first MCP joint)
- De Quervain's tenosynovitis

Fingers

- Inflammatory arthritis
- Osteoarthritis
- Tenosynovitis
- Carpal tunnel syndrome
- Ulnar compression syndromes
- Raynaud's phenomenon (vasospasm)
- Vasculitis

As with most examinations, it is important first to observe. In the rheumatological examination, it is then important to feel the area concerned and then move it.

Outline of the Rheumatological Examination

- Observe
- Touch/palpate
- Move

Much can be gathered from careful observation. In fact, a diagnosis can often be reached even before touching the patient! First look at the hands in general. Look for swelling. Swelling can be difficult to detect so compare sides. It can be confined to one joint or many joints. It can be due to tenosynovitis (inflammation of tendon sheaths). It often involves subcutaneous tissues around the joint. Swelling can be quite diffuse, such as in the RS3PE syndrome (remitting symmetrical seronegative synovitis

Kichu's thoughts . . .

Most common cause of pain at the base of the thumb (first carpometacarpal joint) is osteoarthritis.

The most common cause of pain in a distal interphalangeal joint is osteoarthritis (think of psoriatic arthritis).

When there is swelling of the metacarpophalangeal joints, think of rheumatoid arthritis (but remember hereditary haemochromatosis if it is only the second and third MCP joints).

with peripheral oedema), or quite localized such as in synovitis or tenosynovitis.

Look for muscle wasting, which can be easily seen on the dorsum of the hand (interossei muscles), thenar and hypothenar eminences. Again, compare sides to detect differences. Wasting can be due to disuse or a neurological lesion. Look for dilated veins that occur with inflammation. Look for subcutaneous nodules.

Cause of Subcutaneous Nodules

- Gouty tophi
- Rheumatoid nodules
- Heberden's nodes (technically not a subcutaneous nodule)
- Xanthelasma
- Lipoma
- Calcinosis
- Rheumatic fever
- Sarcoidosis

Look at the shape of the hands. Look for ulnar deviation of the fingers (rheumatoid arthritis). This is due to an erosive arthropathy of the MCP joints that results in ligament and bone destruction resulting in deviation of the fingers. Look for the classic changes of rheumatoid

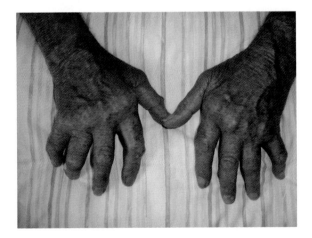

Figure 7.1.   Rheumatoid arthritis.

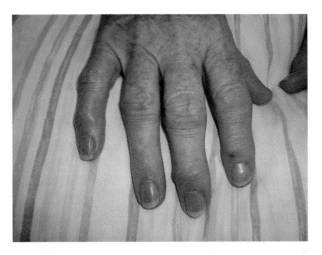

Figure 7.2.   Inspection of the hand.

arthritis — Boutonnière deformity, swan neck deformity and
Z-deformity of the thumb. The patient may be unable to straighten
the fingers. This maybe due to joint disease, but can be due to tightening of the skin seen in scleroderma or contracture of the palmar
aponeurosis (Dupuytren's contracture).

Now look carefully at the fingernails for changes of psoriasis.
There are five nail changes associated with psoriasis — pitting (more
than 20 pits per nail are pathological), ridging, onycholysis, colour
changes and hyperkeratosis. Approximately 10–20% of patients
with psoriasis develop an arthritis. Look also for vasculitic changes
such as splinter haemorrhages. The periungual region may also have
dilated veins. Capillaroscopy is the best method for detecting these.
This requires a capilloscope and is beyond what is expected in a
routine examination. In these circumstances, the pattern of the dilatation is associated with various connective tissue diseases.

Five forms of psoriatic arthritis

1. Inflammatory asymmetrical oligoarthritis
2. Symmetrical inflammatory polyarthritis similar to rheumatoid
   arthritis
3. Psoriatic spondyloarthropathy

4.   Predominantly DIP joint involvement
5.   Arthritis mutilans

Ask the patient to turn his/her hands over. Carefully look for telangiectasia especially in the fingers. Telangiectasia are usually only 1–2 mm in diameter and are due to dilatation of capillaries and venules. These are associated with CREST (Calcinosis, Raynaud's, Esophageal dysmotility, Sclerodactyle and Telengectasia) syndrome. Look for Dupuytren's contractures (due to a thickening of the

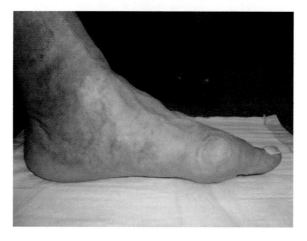

Figure 7.3.   Inspection of the foot.

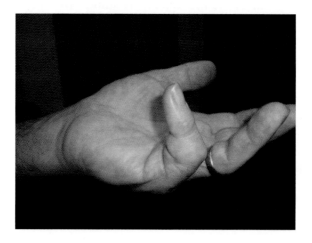

Figure 7.4.   Dupuytren's contractures.

palmar fascia). Consequently, the fingers are flexed at the MCP joints. They are not tender.

CREST syndrome is a limited form of scleroderma. Calcinosis can be seen often on the pulps of the fingers. However, calcinosis can occur anywhere. They are usually small hard white lesions and can be tender. Sclerodactyle is the end result of skin tightening and gives the fingers a tapered appearance. Raynaud's phenomenon and oesophageal dysmotility are usually obtained from the history.

One will occasionally see Raynaud's phenomenon occurring particularly in the colder months. Classically, this begins with the fingers becoming pale or white due to vascular spasm. There is often pain associated with the spasm. The fingers then become cyanotic or blue. Finally, as the spasm resolves, they become flushed or red. With severe Raynaud's phenomenon, the fingertips become ischaemic and form ulcers. The ulcers can be of variable severity. They can become infected with associated cellulitis or paronychia. As the ulcers heal, they often leave a hardened scar like on the fingertip.

Subcutaneous calcinosis can sometimes be difficult to distinguish from gouty tophi. Tophi are usually much larger and less in number than subcutaneous calcinosis. They also occur in close proximity to a joint. Occasionally, chalk-like material (tophus) will exude from the lesion.

Finally it is time to palpate the joints. Each joint must be individually palpated. The clinician needs to know if there is inflammation in the joint. Therefore, the joint is palpated to detect swelling (bony or soft), warmth, synovial thickening, an effusion and tenderness. In the hands, it is often easier to move the joint at the same time as the joint is palpated. The joint can be moved through its range of motion to detect limitations in function.

Cardinal Signs of Inflammation

- Rubor (erythema)
- Calor (heat)
- Dolor (pain)

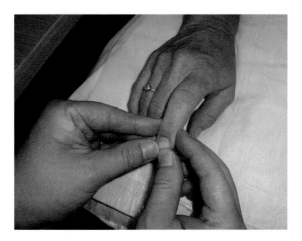

Figure 7.5.   Examination of the hand.

- Tumour (swelling)
- Rigor (stiffness)
- Functio laesa (loss of function)

Begin at the distal interphalangeal (DIP) joints. Palpate the DIP joint by squeezing the joint from opposite sides. Feel for swelling — bony swelling is hard and non-tender. Bony lesions at the DIP joints are Heberden's nodes and are due to osteoarthritis. There is joint space narrowing and osteophyte formation with a subsequent decrease in range of motion. Boggy swelling with tenderness suggests synovitis. Synovitis of the DIP joints is most often due to psoriatic arthritis or gout but can be seen in other forms of inflammatory synovitis.

Examining Hands (DIP, PIP, MCP)

Move onto the proximal interphalangeal (PIP) joints. The joints can be examined in the same way as the DIP joints. Bony, non-tender swelling of the PIP joints are known as Bouchard nodes and are again due to joint space narrowing and osteophyte formation. Boggy swelling and tenderness suggests synovitis. It can be difficult to detect an effusion. Gently squeeze the joint from opposite sides. If

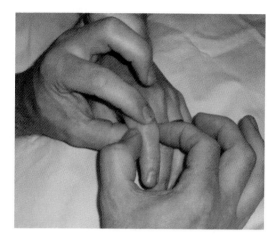

Figure 7.6.   Examination of the hand.

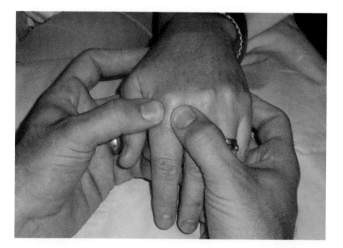

Figure 7.7.   Examination of the metacarpophalangeal joint.

there is an effusion, the examiner will feel a bulge of fluid and the joint margins will become indistinct. Gently move the joint through its range of motion. Osteoarthritis and synovitis will result in a decreased range of motion.

Examine the metacarpophalangeal (MCP) joints next. This time, palpate the joint using your two thumbs with the palm of the patient's hand in your fingers. Feel for synovitis. Again, this can be difficult to detect and needs to be done carefully. Notice if there is a loss of definition between the metacarpal heads due to periarticular swelling. Feel for subluxation by holding the metacarpals still with one hand and grasping the proximal phalanx with the other hand. Gently move the MCP joint and feel for subluxation.

Check for limitation in movement by asking the patient to make a fist. With significant joint disease, the patient will be unable to tuck their fingers into the palm of their hand. As a measure of how much limitation there is, the distance between the middle fingertip and the palm of the hand can be measured. This can then be used as an objective measure of disease progression.

Note any "triggering" of the fingers. This is due to inflammation or a small nodule getting trapped with in the flexor tendon sheath. The patient can flex the finger, but cannot extend them without excessive force or assisting the finger with the other hand. It can occur in isolation or in association with tenosynovitis in inflammatory arthritis such as rheumatoid arthritis or psoriatic arthritis.

The thumb needs special attention. Tenosynovitis commonly involves the thumb and is usually caused by overuse. The abductor pollicis longus and the extensor pollicis brevis sheaths become inflamed resulting in pain made worse by movement. Swelling can

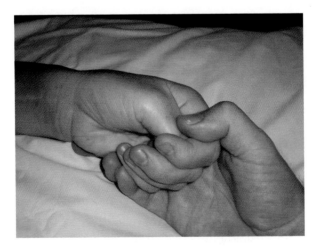

Figure 7.8.   Examination of the hand.

be detected over the radial styloid. To check for this, ask the patient to place their thumb in the palm of their hand (on the same side). Gently move the wrist in an ulnar direction. This test is known as Finkelstein's test. A positive test will cause pain along the line of the tendons. This is known as de Quervain's tenosynovitis. Osteoarthritis of the first carpometacarpal (metacarpotrapezium) joint and scaphotrapezium joint usually gives a negative test. In osteoarthritis, compression of the joint causes pain at the base of the thumb. If the pain is localised to these joints and they are tender to palpation, the pain is probably due to osteoarthritis.

Wrist Pain

The wrist is a complex joint that is difficult to thoroughly examine. It is an ellipsoid joint with the distal radius and triangular fibrocartilage (attached to the distal ulna) at the proximal end and the scaphoid, lunate and triquetrum at the distal end. It has a broad range of movement (80–90° flexion, 70–80° dorsiflexion, 40–50° ulnar deviation and 15–20° radial deviation) yet maintains its stability.

Wrist examination

Initially palpate the wrist joint with the palm down. Palpate the wrist joint in the same manner as examining the MCP joints (use both thumbs with the fingers on the volar aspect supporting the wrist). Feel the ulnar styloid. This is often tender in rheumatoid arthritis due to a combination of synovitis and tenosynovitis. There will be swelling medial to the ulnar styloid with significant tenosynovitis. Feel the radial styloid. Then grasp both styloids with separate hands and attempt to move them in the anteroposterior plane. Pain with this movement is due to disease in the inferior radioulnar joint, which is approximately midway between the two styloid processes.

Feel for swelling in the wrist. This is best felt on the dorsum of the wrist just distal to the distal radioulnar joint. With synovitis, there will be boggy swelling and tenderness. Next, palpate along

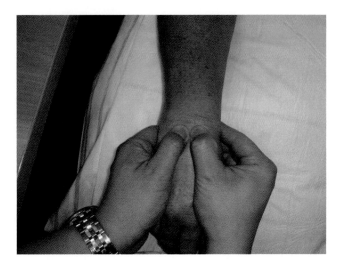

Figure 7.9.   Examination of the wrist.

the joint line towards the ulnar styloid. Common causes of tenderness here are disruption of the triangular fibrocartilage, inflammation of the ulnar collateral ligament or tendonitis of the extensor carpi ulnaris tendon. Then palpate back towards the radial styloid. Localized swelling and superficial tenderness maybe due to inflammation of the extensor compartments. There are six compartments along the dorsum of the wrist. Palpate the anatomical snuffbox. Marked tenderness here suggests a fracture of the scaphoid.

Turn the wrist over. Palpate along the anterior joint line. Tendonitis of the flexor carpi radialis and flexor carpi ulnaris will result in focal tenderness at their respective insertion sites. Test the range of movement of the wrist with passive, then active, movement. The best way to test passive movement is to ask the patient to place the palms of their hands together and then the dorsum of their hands together. Test active movement by asking the patient to extend their wrist and hold it in that position. The examiner then pushes against the extended hand. Similarly test for active flexion by asking the patient to hold the wrist flexed whilst the examiner tries to straighten the wrist.

Wrist Examination

Test for carpal tunnel and ulnar tunnel syndromes. Carpal tunnel syndrome is due to the compression of the median nerve in the carpal tunnel at the wrist. Ulnar tunnel syndrome is due to compression of the ulnar nerve in the ulnar tunnel at the wrist, but is usually compression at the elbow (the "funny bone"). Look for wasting of the thenar and hypothenar eminences. Test for paraesthesia. Pin prick sensation will be reduced on the anterior aspect of the thumb, index, middle and the lateral aspect of the ring fingers in carpal tunnel syndrome. In ulnar nerve compression, the fifth and medial aspect of the ring finger will have decreased pin prick sensation. Test for weakness. Test the strength of the pincer grip between the thumb and index finger. Then test the pincer grip between thumb and fifth finger. Tap over the median nerve. A positive Tinel's sign will cause shooting pains into the fingertips. Then compress the median nerve at the wrist by holding your index finger over the median nerve and flexing the wrist. A positive Phalen's sign will cause pain in the distribution of the median nerve.

Finally, test function of the hand. The pincer grip has already been tested whilst testing for carpal tunnel syndrome. Further functional testing includes use of a key or pen and undoing or doing up a button.

> **Kichu's thoughts . . .**
>
> Pain in the fingers that wakes a patient at night and is relieved by vigorously shaking the hand is often due to carpal tunnel syndrome.

Summary Examination of the Hand and Wrist

- Observe
  - Skin (nails, nodules, rashes)
  - Joints (swelling, deformity)
  - Wasting
- Palpation
  - Examine each joint individually

- Function
- Neurological examination

CASE STUDY 7.2

Thirty-five-year-old male who is a manual labourer presents with an acute onset of elbow pain. He was at work when he felt his elbow getting progressively more painful. There was no injury to the elbow. When he comes and sees you, he has a large swelling on the posterior aspect of the olecranon which is exquisitely tender to touch.

What is your diagnosis?

Elbow Pain

Common causes of elbow pain are usually not due to the joint itself. Most cases are due to localised tendonitis or bursitis. It is uncommon for synovitis to affect the elbow joint in isolation. If there is isolated synovitis, then it is most likely due to infection, gout or psoriatic arthritis.

Causes of elbow pain

- Intra-articular
- Synovitis
- Osteoarthritis
- Loose body
- Periarticular
  - Lateral epicondylitis
  - Medial epicondylitis
  - Bursitis
- Referred
  - Cervical disease
  - Shoulder disease
  - Cardiac ischaemia

Examination begins with careful observation. Position the elbow at 90° on a pillow. Look for swelling over the olecranon. If swollen, it is most likely olecranon bursitis. This is often due to gout, but trauma and infection can look similar. Look for swelling over the lateral and medial epicondyles. These points are the insertion points for the common extensor tendons and flexor tendons of the wrist respectively. Inflammation of these points results in lateral epicondylitis (tennis elbow) and medial epicondylitis (golfer's elbow), respectively. An effusion of the elbow will be seen with swelling between the lateral epicondyle and tip of the olecranon and fullness of the cubital fossa.

Palpate the joint next. Palpate the lateral and medial epicondyles. These will be tender if inflamed. Palpate the olecranon, feeling for a distinct fluid collection due to bursitis. There maybe nodules which should be palpated at the same time.

Rheumatoid nodules are rubbery in texture and usually nontender. Gouty tophi are hard and often show white areas close to the surface. They may also be ulcerated. Other causes of nodules in this location are much less common and include xanthelasma, sarcoidosis, rheumatic nodules and lipomas. Check for joint tenderness

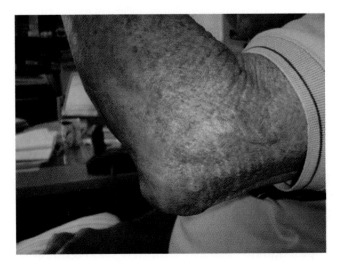

Figure 7.10. Inspection of the elbow.

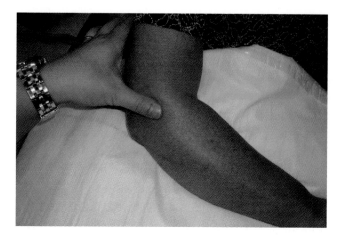

Figure 7.11.   Checking for joint tenderness — elbow.

by palpating between the lateral epicondyle and the tip of the olecranon.

Passive movement should be checked first. Gently move the elbow through its range of motion (40–180°). With an effusion, the elbow will not be able to be fully extended and can be limited in lateral epicondylitis. Hold the elbow at 90° and check for supination and pronation. There should be 180° of rotation. Limitation in movement is due to joint pathology. Pain on pronation can occur with medial epicondylitis and pain with supination can occur with lateral epicondylitis. In patients with hypermobility, extension of the elbow is beyond 0°. This can be part of a hypermobility syndrome (see below).

By now, the examiner should have localised the cause of the elbow pain. Active movements will confirm your clinical suspicion. To test for lateral epicondylitis, check active wrist extension. This is painful with lateral epicondylitis.

Similarly check for medial epicondylitis. Test active flexion. Ask the patient to hold the wrist in flexion and push against the palm of the hand. This will be painful in medial epicondylitis.

Triceps tendonitis and bicipital tendonitis are much less common. Triceps tendonitis will give pain over the olecranon with active extension of the elbow. Bicipital tendonitis will give pain in the middle of the cubital fossa with active elbow flexion.

Hypermobility Syndrome

There are five features to look for on examination when a patient is suspected of having a hypermobility syndrome.

1. The first is to see if the patient can place their thumb on their forearm by flexing the thumb at the wrist. If it is possible, the patient is allocated one point for each thumb. These points are added up to give a final score.
2. Next, ask the patient to hyperextend the fifth finger at the MCP joint. If this is greater then 90° then the patient is allocated one point for each finger.
3. Next, observe extension of the elbow. Extension beyond 0° gives another point for each elbow.
4. Then ask the patient to stand and push their knees into extension. Extension beyond 0° again allocates one point to each knee.
5. Finally, ask the patient to bend forward. If the patient is able to place their hands flat on the ground with their knees extended, they are allocated another point.

A score out of 9 can be given. A score of 4 or more plus three months of arthralgia will fit the criteria for the benign joint hypermobility syndrome. This is a common cause of joint pain especially in younger females.

Shoulder Pain

Shoulder pain is common. Pain can be due to intra-articular causes, periarticular causes and can be referred from other areas, especially the cervical spine. For the purposes of this chapter, it is important to be able to differentiate between a number of common problems outlined below.

Causes of Shoulder Pain

Intra-articular

- Glenohumeral synovitis
- Labral tear
- Glenohumeral osteoarthritis
- Adhesive capsulitis

Periarticular causes

- Rotator cuff tear
- Rotator cuff tendonitis
- Rotator cuff impingement
- Subacromial bursitis
- Polymyalgia rheumatica

Referred pain

- Acromioclavicular joint pathology
- Cervical spine pathology
- Diaphragmatic irritation

Differential Diagnosis of Shoulder Pain: Clinical Signs

Diagnosis	Location of pain	Swelling	Tenderness	Passive movement	Resisted movement
Rotator cuff tendonitis[a]					
• supraspinatus tendonitis	Outer aspect of shoulder	Minimal	Subacromial	Normal but painful abduction	Painful abduction
• infraspinatus tendonitis	Posterior shoulder	Minimal	Posterior shoulder	Normal but painful external rotation	Painful external rotation
• subscapularis tendonitis	Postero-inferior shoulder	Minimal		Normal but painful internal rotation	Painful internal rotation
Bicipital tendonitis	Anterior, may radiate down arm	Minimal	Bicipital groove	Pain stretching the tendon	Painful elbow and shoulder flexion
Capsulitis					
• early phase	Deep in shoulder	Minimal	Upper trapezius	Pain at limits	Mostly normal
• late phase	Deep in shoulder but less intense	Minimal	Minimal	Markedly diminished in all directions	Mostly normal
Acromio-clavicular joint	Over acromio-clavicular joint	Superiorly with effusion	In the joint	Pain with abduction	Normal
Glenohumeral joint	Anterior or posterior	Anterior with effusion	Anterior or posterior	Decreased pain with synovitis	Normal
Subacromial bursitis[b]	Outer aspect of shoulder	Laterally	Laterally	Decreased abduction due to pain	Normal

[a] Rotator cuff tears have the same signs as for tendonitis. However, there is often wasting of the affected muscle and significant weakness.

[b] There is often associated supraspinatus tendonitis with subacromial bursitis, which results in mixed signs.

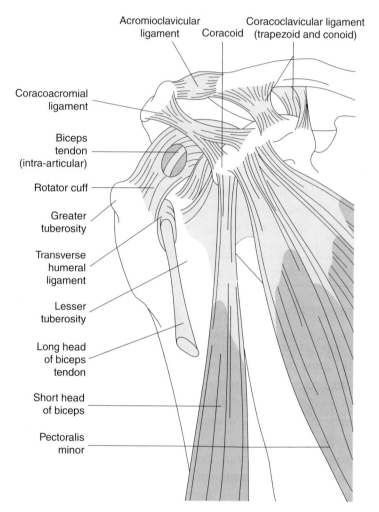

LIGAMENTOUS AND MUSCULOTENDINOUS ATTACHMENTS ABOUT THE SHOULDER JOINT

Acromioclavicular ligament

Coracoid

Coracoclavicular ligament (trapezoid and conoid)

Coracoacromial ligament

Biceps tendon (intra-articular)

Rotator cuff

Greater tuberosity

Transverse humeral ligament

Lesser tuberosity

Long head of biceps tendon

Short head of biceps

Pectoralis minor

Figure 7.12.   Ligamentous and musculotendinous attachments about the shoulder joint.

This will seem overwhelming initially. However, with an understanding of the anatomy, the signs become easy to interpret (Figure 7.12).

Examination of the shoulder begins with exposing the area. Ask the patient to remove outer garments. This may be difficult for the patient to do due to the shoulder problem (and this should be noted by the examiner!). Inspect from anterior, lateral and posterior aspects. Look for swelling and wasting. Wasting can be subtle so the shoulder should be compared to the opposite shoulder.

Begin palpation by standing behind the patient. Place your hand over the shoulder and feel for warmth. Palpate the inferior to the lateral end of the spine of the scapula with your thumb. This is the posterior aspect of the glenohumeral joint. Tenderness suggests glenohumeral disease. Then palpate laterally under the acromion. Tenderness here is due to subacromial bursitis or supraspinatus tendonitis. Next palpate anteriorly with your index and middle fingers. Feel in the bicipital groove for bicipital tendonitis. Feel just medial to the coracoid process for anterior glenohumeral joint tenderness. Finally palpate the acromioclavicular joint. This is approximately 2 cm medial to the tip of the acromion.

Passive movements should be carried out from behind the patient. Stabilize the scapula by placing your fingers on the spine of the scapula and your thumb on the inferior angle of the scapula. With the elbow extended abduct the arm. A painful arc occurs when there is impingement of the supraspinatus tendon. Initially with abduction there is enough space for the supraspinatus tendon in the subacromial space but as the arm is abducted further the space narrows. This results in impingement and pain. This usually begins at approximately 70° abduction. Pain continues until 120° abduction. At this point the pain is relieved, as once again there is space for the supraspinatus tendon.

The subacromial bursa and biceps tendon can also become impinged. With subacromial bursitis, the painful arc tends to occur earlier than with supraspinatus tendonitis and there is no relief of pain above 120° abduction. In fact, it is usually too painful to continue the abduction. Subacromial bursitis and supraspinatus tendonitis often occur together, so the clinical signs can be mixed.

With the biceps tendon, the impingement occurs with abduction when the shoulder is flexed approximately 20° and then abducted. Abduction is also painful with acromioclavicular joint disease.

Causes of a monoarthritis of the acromioclavicular joint are the same as for peripheral joints. However, a tender joint without an effusion is usually due to osteoarthritis. With synovitis of the gleno-humeral joint, all movements are painful.

Causes of Monoarthritis

- Inflammatory synovitis (e.g. rheumatoid arthritis, psoriatic arthritis)
- Infection
- Gout
- Pseudogout
- Osteoarthritis
- Haemarthrosis
- Avascular necrosis
- Stress fracture
- Malignancy
- Pigmented villonodular synovitis

Test for extension. With the arm by the side and elbow extended, bring the arm back. Anterior shoulder pain occurs with biceps tendonitis.

Test for internal and external rotation. With the arm by the patient's side and the elbow flexed to 90°, rotate the arm towards the abdomen and then laterally. The hand should be able to touch the abdomen. Normal external rotation is 60–80° (compare to the normal side, however with rotator cuff disease, the problem is often bilateral). Then ask the patient to put their hand behind their back and see how far they can move their thumb up their spine. The vertebral level should be noted. External rotation (as well as other movements) is severely limited in capsulitis.

Now move on to testing resisted movements. Again from behind, check for resisted abduction. Ask the patient to abduct the arm against resistance. Immediate pain suggests supraspinatus tendonitis as the supraspinatus is the muscle used during the first 20° of abduction.

Weakness implies a tear or partial tear of the supraspinatus tendon. Then, ask the patient to raise the arm to 90° abduction and again test resistance. Weakness suggests deltoid weakness, which can be due to shoulder pathology or a sign of more global proximal weakness.

Then move to the front of the patient. Ask the patient to leave their arm by their side, flex the elbow to 90° and their wrist in a neutral position. Place your hand against the patient's hand. Test resisted internal rotation by asking the patient to push against your hand. Pain suggests subscapularis tendonitis and weakness suggests a rupture or partial rupture of the tendon.

Test for resisted external rotation. Place your hand against the back of the patient's hand. Ask the patient to push with the back of their hand against your hand. Pain suggests infraspinatus tendonitis and weakness suggests rupture or partial rupture of the infraspinatus tendon.

Often when examining the shoulder, the signs that are elicited are mixed. This is because often more than one structure is involved. For instance, in supraspinatus tendonitis there is often involvement of the subacromial bursa or biceps tendon. Consequently, the signs will be somewhat mixed and difficult to interpret. Therefore, if a particular lesion is suspected, then further tests should be carried out to confirm the initial signs.

Lower Back Pain

Lower back pain is a very common complaint. The lifetime prevalence of an episode of lower back pain is 80%. Many of these episodes are relatively transient in nature and the exact cause of the pain will never be known. However, there are important causes of back pain that need to be identified. History is extremely important. There are so-called "red flags" that need to be identified. "Red flags" suggest that there is a important and possibly malignant cause for the back pain. These usually require further investigation. Similarly, there are "yellow flags" that need to be identified.

The examination of the lower back usually begins with the patient sitting in a chair. Note if the patient is sitting comfortably or whether they are in pain. Ask the patient to stand from the chair. If they require the arm rests to stand up, then ask the patient to try again, but not to use the arm rests this time. An inability to do this is suggestive of proximal muscle weakness (consider myositis or spinal canal stenosis), but can also be due to severe lower back pain.

Red flags in back pain

- History of malignancy
- Age over 50
- Fever
- Weight loss
- Night pain
- Bladder or bowel disturbance
- History of trauma (especially minor)
- Failure to improve with treatment

Yellow flags in back pain

- Identify psychosocial and occupational factors that may increase the risk of chronicity in acute LBP
- Attitudes and beliefs about pain
- Behaviours
- Compensation issues
- Diagnostic and treatment issues
- Emotions
- Family
- Work circumstances

Causes of Back Pain

- Bone disease
- Fracture
  - Malignancy
  - Scheuermann's disease

- o Osteomyelitis
- o Myelofibrosis
- Paget's disease
- Osteoid osteoma and other primary bone tumours
- Zygapophyseal joint disease
  - o Osteoarthritis
- Autoimmune
  - o Spondyloarthropathy e.g. ankylosing spondylitis
- Neurological
  - o Nerve root compression
  - o Spinal canal stenosis
- Intervertebral disc herniation
- Diffuse idiopathic skeletal hyperostosis (DISH)
- Referred
  - o Endometriosis
  - o Aortic aneurysm
  - o Retroperitoneal fibrosis
  - Non-specific lower back pain

Ask the patient to stand with their back towards the examiner. Look carefully at the back. Look for a scoliosis, loss of lumbar lordosis (think ankylosing spondylitis) or kyphosis (think compression fractures).

Next, palpate the spine. Initially palpate from the lower thoracic vertebrae towards the sacrum. Palpate each vertebral body individually for tenderness. Palpate the sacrum then palpate the sacro-iliac joints. These are best felt below the dimples of Venus. Next, palpate the paraspinal muscles for tenderness and spasm. Palpate along the posterior iliac crest for muscle tenderness and spasm.

Test spinal movements. Begin with forward flexion. Ask the patient to keep their knees extended and to try and touch the ground. With hypermobility, the patient will be able to place their hands flat on the ground. With disease of the lower spine, there is limitation of flexion. The distance between the floor and the fingertips should be noted. This can then be used to monitor disease progression. Test lateral flexion. Ask the patient to slide their hand down the outside of their leg. Their fingertip should be able to reach the lower aspect of the patella. With nerve root compression, the patient will often have pain down the leg on the same side as the lateral flexion.

Test extension. Stand behind the patient and ask the patient to lean back. This often accentuates nerve root compression. Ask the patient to stand straight again. Then ask the patient to keep their feet in one spot and rotate 45°, then ask the patient to lean back. Pain that is elicited in the lumbar spine is suggestive of zygapophyseal joint disease. Do this again with the patient rotated in the opposite direction.

A more objective measure of lumbar flexion is with the Schober's test (Figure 7.13). With the patient standing, place a tape measure along their lumbar spine. Mark a position 10 cm above the level of the dimples of Venus. Firmly hold the tape measure at the distal end of the spine. Ask the patient to flex forward with their knees extended. At maximal flexion, the 10 cm mark should be at least 15 cm.

Test quickly for muscle weakness. Ask the patient to stand on their toes. Inability to do this suggests calf weakness, which could be a L5 or S1 nerve root lesion. Ask the patient to stand on their heels. Patients are often unsteady, but a foot drop will be obvious.

The patient must then be assessed for a specific nerve lesion. The neurological examination of the lower limb is covered elsewhere.

SCHOBER TEST

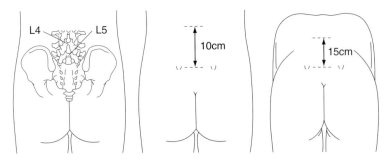

Figure 7.13.   Schober test to measure ability to flex the lumbar spine.

The Hip and Sacroiliac Joints

Patients often present with "hip pain" as their main complaint. "Hip pain" often means different pain to different people. It is important to localize the location of the pain. Often the pain is over the lumbar spine or sacroiliac joint. The pain can be over the greater trochanter and radiate down the outer aspect of the leg. This is usually trochanteric bursitis or gluteus medius tendonitis. Hip joint pain is a deep pain over the anterior aspect of the hip that radiates into the groin. However, 20% of the time it can be felt into the thigh, the buttock or radiate down to the knee.

Sacroiliac joint pain is also a deep pain. It is often made worse by sitting and relieved by standing. The pain is usually over the sacroiliac joint. In sacroilitis, the pain can move from one buttock to the other. There is usually associated stiffness, particularly in the morning and after periods of immobility ("gelling").

Examination of these joints is best done together. Begin the examination by inspecting the hip and surrounding structures. With the patient standing, look for wasting of the glutei or quadriceps muscles. Look for a fixed deformity. The most common is a flexed

---

CASE STUDY 7.3

Mr. MC is 21 years old. Over the last five years, Mr. MC has had intermittent lower back pain. This usually comes in "flairs" that can last for a week at a time, but sometimes it lasts for months. When he has a "flair", he has significant difficulty getting out of bed in the morning and it isn't until he has had a hot shower that he feels like he can move freely.

The stiffness is usually in the buttock region. He also notices that if he sits still for more than 30 minutes, he again gets stiffness in the lower spine that makes it difficult to get moving.

Examination shows a decrease in lower spinal movements.

What is your differential diagnosis?

and laterally rotated position as this is the most comfortable position for the patient with a hip problem. Fixed flexion deformities can be masked by the patient increasing their pelvic tilt. This results in an increase in lumbar lordosis.

Examine the patient's gait next. Observe their gait from the front, side and from behind. There are four patterns to observe:

1. **Antalgic gait.** This is caused by a painful hip. The patient tries to minimise the time spent weight bearing on the painful hip.
2. **Trendelenburg gait.** This occurs when there is weakness of the hip abductors due to an unstable hip. With a normal gait, the hip abductors contract when the weight is borne on the same side. In a Trendelenburg gait, there is weakness of the abductors. This results in the pelvis tilting in the wrong direction when the patient is asked to stand on one leg. The observer will see the "sound side sag" (see below). If there is weakness on both sides, the patient will have a waddling gait.
3. **Swinging gait.** The whole leg is swung around. This can be due to ankylosis of the hip joint or due to a hemiplegia.
4. **Adductor gait.** This results in scissoring of the legs, due to a muscle adductor spasm. This is usually due to bilateral hip disease.

Test Hip Movements

Active and passive movements need to be tested. This is best done with the patient lying supine. Test first for passive movements. Test flexion by grasping the ipsilateral tibia with one hand and placing the other hand on the opposite anterior superior iliac spine (ASIS). Push the tibia forward. Flexion is usually limited by the thigh coming into contact with the anterior abdominal wall (approximately 140°).

Test internal and external rotation. Flex the hip and knee to 90°. With one hand on the knee and another holding onto the ankle, turn the hip joint by moving the ankle towards the opposite hip (tests external rotation) and then move the ankle in the opposite direction (tests internal rotation). It always seems counterintuitive that moving the foot medially tests external rotation and vice versa! Normal range is 60° of external rotation and 30° of internal rotation.

Test for abduction. Again, one hand must be on the opposite ASIS to the hip being tested. Hold the lower leg and gently abduct the hip joint. Feel for movement in the pelvis. Once the pelvis starts to move, this is the limit of abduction. Normal range is 45°. Then check adduction by bringing the leg across the contralateral leg. Normal adduction is to 25°.

Extension is tested with the patient in the prone position. Again, steady the pelvis by placing one hand on the posterior pelvic crest. Passively extend the hip by lifting the leg from the thigh. Normal movement is to 15°.

Active movements are best done with the patient standing. There is a wide range of normal movement, particularly in flexion.

Thomas' Test

This test is designed to detect a fixed flexion deformity of the hip. The idea is to abolish the lumbar lordosis and look for flexion in the hip. To abolish the lordosis, the examiner fully flexes the contralateral hip. The contralateral hip is then slowly brought back to the neutral position. When the lumbar spine starts to become elevated from the bed, stop lowering the contralateral leg. Take note of the position of the hip being tested. If there is a fixed flexion deformity, the hip will be in a flexed position.

Trendelenburg Test

Trendelenburg described a test that was able to assess hip abductor function. A positive test suggested hip joint pathology, especially congenital dislocation of the hip and progressive muscular atrophy. It was particularly useful prior to the use of X-rays. It does have false positive results (due to pain, lack of cooperation from the patient and due to impingement between the iliac crest and rib cage) especially if done incorrectly.

The normal function of the hip involves contraction of the hip abductors when weight is transferred to the same side. This allows the pelvis to remain level. When there is disease of the hip, there is often associated weakness of the hip abductors.

Performing the test properly takes time and full cooperation from the patient. To perform the test, ask the patient to stand on both feet. Observe the pelvic rims from behind. They should be level.

Ask the patient to raise the leg on the side not being tested, with the hip held at approximately 30° flexion. The position of the pelvic rim is again noted. The patient can be supported by holding their shoulders. The patient is then asked to raise the non-stance side of the pelvis as high as possible and maintain it for 30 seconds.

A negative test (or normal response) is when the pelvic rim remains elevated. A positive test (or abnormal result) is when the pelvic rim doesn't remain elevated, but sags. It is also felt to be positive if the elevation can't be maintained for 30 seconds (a delayed response). Therefore, the *sound side sags*.

Significance of the Trendelenburg test

Neurological weakness of abduction	Grade 5/5 strength is needed for a normal response
Mechanical disorders: Congenital dislocation of the hip	Always positive
Subluxation of the hip	Usually positive (delayed response)
Coxa vara	Usually positive
Perthes' disease	Usually negative
Arthritis of the hip	Variable response
Fractured neck of femur	Usually positive
Avascular necrosis of the hip	Usually positive
Spinal disorders: Ankylosing spondylitis	Negative unless there is also hip involvement
Spinal kyphosis	Does not affect the result
Spinal scoliosis	May give a false positive result due to the lower costal margin coming into contact with the iliac crest
Spinal nerve root impingement	May cause a false positive

Causes of hip pain

Intra-articular
- Osteoarthritis
- Infection
- Synovitis
- Labral tear
- Perthes' disease (children)

Periarticular
- Osteonecrosis of the femoral head
- Fractured neck of femur
- Malignancy in femoral head
- Trochanteric bursitis
- Gluteus medius tendonitis
- Polymyalgia rheumatica

Referred
- Sacroiliac joint
- Lower back pain
- Inguinal hernia
- Intra-abdominal pathologies

The Knee

The knee is the largest synovial joint in the body. There are three compartments to the joint: the medial and lateral tibiofemoral compartments and the patellofemoral compartment. It is important to know the anatomy of the joint in order to identify a particular lesion.

Examination of the knee should begin with the patient standing. Ask the patient to stand with their feet slightly apart. Look for a deformity of the knee. A genu varum, genu valgum and fixed flexion deformity should be looked for. A genu varum is

> **Kichu's thoughts . . .**
>
> Varus deformity means that the part of the bone distal to the joint is displaced medially.

often due to damage in the medial compartment of the knee joint resulting in a loss of joint space. This is most commonly due to osteoarthritis. A genu valgum is due to damage in the lateral tibiofemoral compartment resulting in joint space loss. A fixed flexion deformity results in an inability to completely extend the knee or "lock it back" into position.

Ask the patient to lie on the bed. Look carefully at the knee for swelling and quadriceps wasting. A synovial effusion results in swelling into the suprapatellar pouch. This is above and medial to the patella.

A prepatellar bursitis gives swelling over the anterior aspect of the patella. Osgood–Schlatter's disease results in swelling over the tibial tubercle. A Baker's cyst is seen as a swelling behind the knee and is due to an outpouching of the synovium into the popliteal fossa.

Palpate the knee. Feel for warmth by comparing the skin temperature over the knee to the other knee. Feel for tenderness. Each structure needs to be separately palpated.

Begin along the edge of the patella. With inflammation in the knee there is usually tenderness along the patella borders. Palpate along the joint line. This will also be tender with inflammation, but can also be tender with structural damage to the menisci or cartilage. Palpate for the medial and lateral collateral ligaments. The lateral collateral ligament is a band-like structure that is easily felt along the lateral border of the knee joint. The medial collateral ligament is a fan-like structure on the medial aspect of the knee. Palpate the insertion of the patella ligament at the tibia. This is often tender in Osgood–Schlatter's disease.

A large effusion is easily seen, but a smaller effusion can be harder to detect. A patella tap is present if there is a moderate-sized effusion. To elicit a patella tap, the examiner places one hand proximal to the patella with the fingers on one side of the thigh and the thumb on the other. This allows synovial fluid in the suprapatellar pouch to be pushed under the patella. With the index and middle fingers of the other hand, the examiner pushes firmly down on the patella. A positive tap occurs if the examiner feels the patella "tap" against the underlying femoral head.

A small effusion can be found by looking for the bulge sign. The fluid in the knee is moved into the suprapatellar pouch by stroking the medial patella gutter in an upward direction. The left hand is then placed on the thigh proximal to the patella to compress the suprapatellar pouch. If the sign is positive, then fluid moves back into the medial patella gutter causing a bulge.

Active and passive movements are then tested. Ask the patient to fully extend the knee. This should be to a neutral position (0°), but sometimes active hyperextension is possible. Active flexion should be to 140°. Test for passive movements. Passive hyperextension is possible to 5–10°. Passive flexion is tested by holding the patients ankle and pushing the heel towards the buttock. Passive flexion is usually 20° more than active flexion.

The final part of the examinations to test the ligaments and the menisci of the knee.

The medial and lateral collateral ligaments, the anterior cruciate ligament and the posterior cruciate ligaments need to be tested.

Anterior cruciate ligament is tested with three manoeuvres: the Lachman test, anterior draw test and the pivot shift test.

The posterior cruciate ligament is tested with the posterior draw sign and reverse pivot shift.

The collateral ligaments are tested by exerting a lateral force (testing medial collateral ligament) and medial force (testing lateral collateral ligament) to the knee whilst held in 30° flexion.

The menisci are tested by palpating for joint line tenderness and McMurray's test.

CASE STUDY 7.4

Miss JM is a 23-year-old woman who is a keen basketball player. During a game last week, she twisted her knee and felt it give way. Initially, it was painful and she was not able to continue with the game. The knee became swollen over the next few hours.

She has had ongoing swelling and difficulty walking.

How would you assess this patient?

Answer: Miss JM describes a traumatic injury whilst playing a sport. The knee gave way, suggesting a mechanical derangement of the knee. The knee became swollen over a few hours, suggesting a tear in the meniscus, anterior cruciate ligament (ACL) or posterior cruciate ligament (PCL). Immediate swelling would suggest a haemarthrosis.

> **Kichu's thoughts . . .**
>
> **Sensitivity and specificity**
> Sensitivity — remember "**SNOUT**" — when a test is highly Sensitive, then Negative test rules the condition **OUT**.
> Specificity — remember "**SPIN**" — when a test is highly Specific, then a Positive test rules the condition **IN**.

Swelling that was confined to the medial or lateral aspect of the knee would suggest a collateral ligament tear.

When examining the knee, it will be important to identify an ongoing effusion. Tests for ACL or PCL rupture or a meniscal tear should be performed. These can be difficult to do at the best of times. However, when there is a significant effusion, it is even harder.

Miss JM had a positive Lachman test and anterior draw sign, suggesting an ACL rupture.

Sensitivity and specificity

Test	Sensitivity	Specificity
Lachman test	0.87	0.93
Anterior draw test	0.48	0.87
Pivot shift test	0.61	0.97
Joint line tenderness for meniscal pathology	0.76	0.29
McMurray test	0.52	0.97

Causes of Knee Pain

Intra-articular
- Synovitis
- Infection

- Osteoarthritis
- Meniscal tears
- Baker's cyst
- Anterior or posterior cruciate ligament tear

Periarticular

- Collateral ligament tear
- Patellar tendonitis
- Bursitis (prepatellar, infrapatellar, pes anserine)
- Bone disease (fracture, spontaneous osteonecrosis of the knee — SONK)

Referred

- Hip
- Lumbar nerve root compression (usually L3)

Causes of Swelling of the Ankle

Articular

- Synovitis
- Infection
- Osteoarthritis

Periarticular

- Tendonitis (Achilles, posterior tibialis)
- Ligament tear or sprain
- Retrocalcaneal bursitis
- Rheumatoid nodule
- Gouty tophus

Systemic
- Peripheral oedema

Palpate the joint by supporting the joint with your fingers and using your thumbs to palpate. Palpate the bony prominences for tenderness. Palpate along the anterior joint line (between the malleoli) for synovitis. Palpate along the line of the tendons for evidence of tendonitis and at the insertion of the Achilles tendon. Finally, palpate the retrocalcaneal bursa.

To check passive movements, have the patient in the supine position with the knee extended. Hold the lower leg with the left hand proximal to the ankle joint. Hold the foot with the right hand just proximal to the midtarsal joints. This will then localise movements in the ankle. Normal dorsiflexion is 15–25° and plantar flexion 40–50°.

There are a number of manoeuvres that can be done to check the ligaments of the ankle. To describe them all is beyond the scope of this chapter; however, the anterior draw test should be done. This is to check the integrity of the anterior talofibular ligament. The examiner holds the anterior aspect of the lower leg with one hand and the posterior heel with the other. The heel is then pulled towards the examiner. If there is excessive forward movement (greater than 3 mm), this suggests a rupture of the anterior talofibular ligament.

Check active movements next. Most movement in the ankle is in the plane of plantar flexion and dorsiflexion. However, in maximal plantar flexion, there is also some inversion. Be careful though because most of the inversion is actually done in the subtalar joints discussed later.

Finally, test resisted movements. Dorsiflexion is done mostly by tibialis anterior. Tendonitis or a tear in the muscle will result in painful dorsiflexion. Weakness without pain is suggestive of a neurological condition (commonly L5 nerve root lesion or common peroneal nerve). Plantar flexion is then tested. It can be difficult to assess mild weakness. The most sensitive test is to ask the patient to stand on their toes. Pain is usually due to a gastrocnemius tear or Achilles tendonitis. Painless weakness can be due to a S1 nerve root lesion.

Ankle Joint

Examination of the ankle joint begins with careful inspection. With the patient standing and then lying, inspect for swelling. An effusion is seen anteriorly and posteriorly to the malleoli. An anterior effusion is seen as a bulge anteriorly between the two malleoli. With an extensive effusion, the swelling extends over the malleoli. A posterior effusion is seen as a swelling between the malleoli and the Achilles tendon. Look for skin changes such as ulcers.

Other causes of swelling around the ankle need to be considered.

Tendonitis causes swelling around the affected tendon. Achilles tendonitis, tibialis posterior tendonitis (lies behind the medial malleolus) and peroneal tendonitis (lie behind the lateral malleolus) need to be identified. Tenosynovitis tends to give a linear swelling rather than a more focal swelling of synovitis.

Ligament sprains of the ankle are one of the most common sporting injuries. The main injuries are to the anterolateral ligaments. These are made up of three ligaments. The weakest is the anterior talofibular ligament. Damage to this results in swelling over the anterolateral aspect of the ankle joint (just medial to the lateral malleolus). The second component is the fibulocalcaneal ligament. Damage here causes swelling inferior to the lateral malleolus. The third component is the posterior talofibular ligament. Damage to this ligament is uncommon, but results in swelling posterior to the lateral malleolus.

A localised cause of swelling around the ankle to consider is retrocalcaneal bursitis. The bursa is located posterior to the insertion of the Achilles tendon. With bursitis, there will be swelling and redness of the skin over this area. Rheumatoid nodules or gouty tophi can also cause localized swellings.

Finally, always consider general oedema as a cause of ankle swelling, so a quick inspection of the other ankle is important.

The Rest of the Foot

There are three main joint regions to be examined — the subtalar joint, the mid-tarsal joints and the toes (metatarsophalangeal joints and interphalangeal joints).

Inspection should be done first and this should encompass the entire foot. Ask the patient to stand. The foot should be examined from behind and from the side. Look for deformity. The Achilles tendon and calcaneus should be in direct alignment. If the calcaneus has moved laterally, then this is a valgus deformity of the hind foot and if the calcaneus has moved medially, then this is a varus deformity of the hind foot.

Next look at the arch of the foot. Lowering of the longitudinal arch is pes planus (flat foot) and elevation is pes cavus.

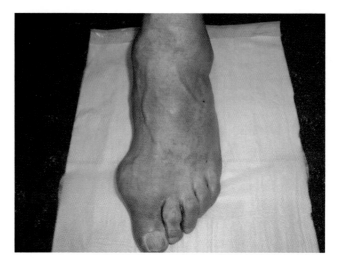

Figure 7.14.   Inspection of the foot.

Look for deformity of the toes. Hallux valgus refers to lateral deviation of the first toe with an angle of greater than 10° at the metatarsophalangeal joint. Other deformities include a mallet toe, hammer toe and claw toe (see diagram).

Look for skin changes which include rashes, ulcers, callus (thickening of the skin due to repetitive irritation), nodules and nail changes.

Look for swelling. Swelling maybe localised to a joint, tendon sheath, bursa or digit. "Sausage digits" occur in a similar fashion to that in the fingers.

Finally, if it is possible, the patient's shoes should be inspected for unequal wear, particularly at the heel.

The Subtalar Joint

The subtalar joint is important for stability of the foot and ability to compensate for circumstances such as uneven ground whilst walking or running. The joint can't be palpated. Swelling in the joint can be seen laterally half way between the lateral malleolus and the heel.

The normal range of movement is 30° of supination (which is a combination of inversion, adduction and plantar flexion) and 20° of pronation (which is a combination of eversion, abduction and dorsi-flexion). The best way to examine this is to grasp the heel with one hand whilst stabilising the ankle with the other hand. Supinate and pronate the joint.

The Mid-Tarsal Joints

The two main joints in this region are the talonavicular joint and calcaneocuboid joints. There are also the intercuneiform joints and tarsometatarsal joints.

Swelling in these joints is easily seen overlying the joint. Palpate the joint for tenderness and warmth. The best way to palpate these joints is by using the thumbs on the dorsal surface whist the fingers support the plantar surface of the foot.

It is difficult to test the individual movements of these joints. With one hand, stabilise the talus and calcaneus and with the other grasp the forefoot. Test for inversion (30°), eversion (20°), pronation and supination. When the foot is maximally pronated, ask the patient to actively supinate the foot. This is done via tibialis anterior and tibialis posterior. Pain with this movement suggests tendonitis or rupture of these muscles.

The Metatarsophalangeal and Interphalangeal Joints

Swelling of the joints can be difficult to detect. Careful observation is required. Swelling in the first metatarsophalangeal joint is usually seen medially and on the dorsal surface. Swelling of the other metatarsophalangeal joints is seen on the dorsal surface. Look for redness over the joint.

Palpate each of these joints individually. Feel for warmth. Place two thumbs on the dorsal aspect of the joint and support the plantar surface with the fingers. Feel for swelling and tenderness.

Both active and passive movements are tested. Passive movement of the first metatarsophalangeal joint has 90° of extension and 45° of flexion. The other metatarsophalangeal joints have 40° of extension and 40° of flexion.

Causes of Pain in Small Joints of the Feet

Articular

- Synovitis
- Osteoarthritis (especially first MTP, dorsal aspect mid-tarsal joints)
- Gout (especially first MTP)

Periarticular

- Plantar fasciitis
- Achilles tendonitis
- Corns, calluses
- Retrocalcaneal bursitis
- Bunion
- Stress fracture of metatarsal bone

Neurological

- L4, L5 or S1 nerve root compression
- Peripheral nerve lesion
- Tarsal tunnel syndrome
- Morton's neuroma

Vascular insufficiency

Summary of the Rheumatological Examination

History taking

Often, the diagnosis or a short differential diagnosis can be made from a careful history. It is important to know which joints are affected and their distribution. Systemic features should be sought.

General inspection

Look at the overall condition of the patient. Look for generalised wasting, Cushingoid features, generalised difficulty in movement and body habitus such as spinal kyphosis. Take note of any devices or aids that the patient may have such as wrist braces or walking sticks. The patient may have a bottle of water to help with their sicca symptoms (dry mouth) even though carrying a bottle of water is a very common thing in the younger individuals.

Face

Have a good look at the patient's face. This will help establish some rapport with the patient. Look for skin tightness (scleroderma), rashes (SLE, scleroderma), Cushingoid features (excessive corticosteroids), hair loss, tophi on the ears, inflammation in the eyes (episcleritis) or parotid swelling (Sjogren's syndrome, sarcoidosis).

Individual joint examination

In a general examination, it is important to identify which joints are problematic. Each peripheral joint should be inspected and palpated. The main features to look for are swelling, redness and deformity. Palpate for tenderness and warmth. Once a joint or series of joints are identified, they can be examined in more detail as outlined in this chapter.

Systemic examination

If a diffuse autoimmune disease is suspected, then an examination of other organ systems is important. Lung disease is common in rheumatoid arthritis and scleroderma. Neurological involvement is seen in Wegener's granulomatosis and polyarteritis nodosa. Inflammatory bowel disease and psoriasis are associated with an inflammatory arthritis. Cardiovascular disease is an important cause of mortality in SLE and rheumatoid arthritis.

X-rays and serological investigations

Before ordering these tests, a clear differential diagnosis should be formulated. These tests will help differentiate between the differential diagnoses or confirm a clinical suspicion.

Features to Look For on Examination of Various Diseases

Rheumatoid arthritis

Hands

- Ulnar deviation and subluxation of MCPs
- Radial deviation and subluxation at the wrist
- Boutonniere and Swan-neck deformity of the fingers
- Z-deformity of the thumb
- Tenosynovitis
- Rupture of tendons
- Nodules
- Vasculitic skin changes
- Wasting of interossei muscles
- Synovitis of PIP, MCP and wrist joints

Elbow

- Nodules
- Olecranon bursitis
- Fixed flexion deformity
- Synovitis

Shoulder

- Wasting of shoulder girdle
- Tenosynovitis
- Synovitis

Acromioclavicular joint

- Synovitis

Temporomandibular joint

- Synovitis

Cervical spine

- Decreased range of motion
- Subluxation (late disease)

Sternoclavicular joint

- Synovitis

Hip
- Quadriceps and gluteal wasting
- Synovitis
- Secondary osteoarthritis

Knee
- Effusion
- Baker's cyst
- Secondary osteoarthritis

Ankle
- Synovitis
- Achilles tendonitis

Hindfoot
- Synovitis
- Valgus deformity and secondary collapse of the longitudinal arch (late disease)

Forefoot
- Synovitis of MTPs
- Dorsal subluxation of proximal phalanges
- Ulcers particularly under metatarsal heads
- Venous disease
- Geodes

Systemic manifestations

Respiratory
- Bibasal fibrosis
- Pleural effusion

Cardiovascular
- Biventricular failure
- Constrictive pericarditis
- Peripheral vascular disease
- Chronic venous congestion

Gastrointestinal
- Felty's syndrome (splenomegaly)

Neurological

- Entrapment neuropathies (especially carpal tunnel syndrome, ulnar compression at the elbow, tarsal tunnel syndrome)
- Peripheral neuropathy
- Atlantoaxial subluxation (long tract signs)

Ocular

- Keratoconjunctivitis sicca
- Scleromalacia
- Episcleritis

Skin

- Nodules
- Ulcers (especially lower leg)
- Vasculitis
- Anaemia (chronic disease)

Complications of Medications

Non-steroidal anti-inflammatory drugs

- Rashes
- Hypertension
- Peptic ulcer disease

Methotrexate

- Oral ulcers
- Anaemia
- Pneumonitis
- Hepatic fibrosis with signs of chronic liver disease

Corticosteroids

- Thin skin
- Easy bruising
- Proximal myopathy
- Abnormal fat distribution (buffalo hump, moon facies)
- Evidence of fracture (e.g. thoracic kyphosis)
- Cataracts
- Hypertension
- Evidence for diabetes

Leflunamide

- Peripheral neuropathy
- Hypertension
- Anaemia
- Malnutrition (chronic diarrhoea)

Gold

- Pneumonitis
- Peripheral neuropathy
- Discolouration of the skin (metallic)
- Corneal deposits

TNF antagonists

- Injection site reactions
- Reactivation of tuberculosis

Systemic Lupus Erythematosis (SLE)

Cutaneous

- "Butterfly" rash
- Discoid lesions
- Panniculitis/vasculitis
- Raynaud's phenomenon

Joint

- Inflammatory synovitis (if this results in a deforming arthritis of the MCP joints it is known as Jaccoud arthropathy)

Oral

- Mouth ulcers

Respiratory

- Pleuritic rub
- Pneumonitis

Cardiac

- Endocarditis (Libman–Sacks lesions)
- Ischaemic heart disease

Muscle

- Myositis

Renal

- Various manifestations from acute renal failure to chronic renal failure. Look for nephrotic syndrome

Neurological

- Cerebrovascular accidents
- Seizures
- Transverse myelitis
- Peripheral neuropathy
- Retinopathy (cytoid bodies)
- Psychosis

Psoriatic Arthritis

Cutaneous

- Nail changes (see text)
- Typical lesions on extensor surfaces of joints (especially elbows and knees), hairline and natal cleft

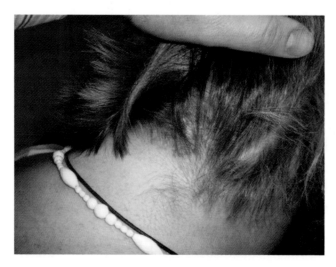

Figure 7.15.   Psoriasis of scalp.

Joint

- Rheumatoid-like distribution
- Inflammatory DIP joint pattern
- Spondyloarthritic pattern
- Inflammatory oligoarthritis
- Arthritis mutilans

Systemic Sclerosis

Cutaneous

There are three phases in the course of the skin disease — the initial inflammatory oedematous phase, an indurative phase and later an atrophic phase.

Oedematous phase — puffiness of the fingers with a loss of normal skin creases. Reduced sweating and oiliness of the skin resulting in drying and fissuring of the skin. There may be digital ulceration due to Raynaud's phenomena and tapering of the fingertips, as well as Paronychia around the nail beds. Look for telangiectasia and subcutaneous calcinosis.

The indurative and atrophic phase results in progressive fibrosis of the skin. There is tightening and thickening of the skin. This can involve the extremities, chest, abdomen, neck and face. If severe, there is an expressionless face, pinching of the skin around the nose and prominence of the frontal teeth due to perioral skin tightening.

Crest

- Syndrome changes (see text)

Joints

- There can be a polysynovitis similar to rheumatoid arthritis

Muscles

- Friction rubs due to fibrin deposition in tendon sheaths
- Muscle atrophy due to decreased joint function (due to skin tightening), myositis or complication of treatment (d-penicillamine, corticosteroids, hydroxychloroquine)

Gastrointestinal
- Small oral aperture and dry mucous membranes
- Signs of swallowing difficulty
- Signs of malnutrition

Hepatic
- Rarely involved, but has been associated with primary biliary cirrhosis; therefore, check for jaundice

Pulmonary
- Lung involvement is nearly universal
- Interstitial fibrosis
- Pulmonary vascular disease (pulmonary hypertension)

Cardiac
- Pericarditis
- Arrhythmias
- Biventricular failure
- Pulmonary hypertension
- Myocarditis

Renal
- Scleroderma renal crisis (may present with typical signs malignant hypertension such as headache, altered vision, heart failure, confusion, seizures)

Neurological
- Trigeminal neuralgia
- Depression

Ankylosing Spondylitis

Joints
- Sacroiliitis
- Peripheral arthritis
- Enthesitis

Eyes
- Uveitis

Cardiac
- Aortic insufficiency
- Heart block

Pulmonary
- Interstitial lung disease (however this is frequently subclinical)

Sjogren's Syndrome

Eyes
- Pericorneal injection due to dryness (can be quantified with a Schirmer's test)

Oral
- Xerostomia (dry mouth)
- Dental caries

Glands
- Parotid gland enlargement
- Salivary gland enlargement

Joints
- Non-erosive synovitis

Cutaneous
- Raynaud's phenomenon
- Vasculitis

Other organ involvement is less common. The major complication is lymphoma, so an abdominal examination and examination of peripheral lymph nodes is required.

Polymyalgia Rheumatica

Polymyalgia is characterised by stiffness and, to a lesser extent, pain involving the proximal hip and shoulder girdles. It is usually worse in the morning, but when it is severe can last all day. Both shoulder and hip girdle symptoms should be present to confirm the diagnosis. It rarely occurs in patients under the age of 50 years old.

Examination will show a generalised stiffness of shoulder and hip movements. Ten percent of patients will have an inflammatory arthritis that is usually in a rheumatoid arthritis like pattern. Alternatively, rheumatoid arthritis can present as polymyalgia rheumatica, but over time, the synovitis will become more prominent, confirming the diagnosis of rheumatoid arthritis.

Giant Cell Arteritis

Giant cell arteritis refers to a vasculitis of the large proximal arteritis that result in the formation of "giant cells" in the wall of the inflamed artery. The condition is also known as temporal arteritis as the temporal arteries are often affected.

It is an important condition to recognize early. Delayed treatment can result in an acute onset of blindness which is often irreversible. The patient will describe headache, scalp tenderness ("Is it painful to brush your hair?"), jaw pain ("Is it painful to chew your food?" or " Does your jaw get tired when you chew food?") or

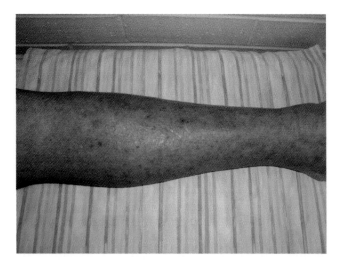

Figure 7.16.   Drug rash from medication.

difficulty swallowing. Occasionally, patients describe pain at the back of the scalp or even ringing in the ear. Often, there are relatively few symptoms.

Diagnosis should include measurements of inflammatory markers and temporal artery biopsy.

If a diagnosis is suspected, the patient should immediately be started on prednisone 1 mg/kg/day.

chapter | 8

Examination of the Vascular System

Arvind Deshpande

Symptoms and signs of vascular disorders are a reflection of multiple vascular occlusive processes affecting target organs. Some of these may be readily apparent as gangrene of a toe along with the absence of a popliteal or a femoral pulse. On the other hand, renal artery stenosis or mesenteric occlusive lesions may remain "silent" or express themselves as hypertension or postprandial pain.

A vascular examination is not complete unless co-morbidities are identified and assessed. The patient's cardiac, pulmonary and renal reserve and his quality of life prior to the vascular

> **Kichu's thoughts . . .**
>
> A palpable pulse in the neck does not mean the internal carotid artery is patent.

event have an important bearing on therapy. The risk-benefit ratio of vascular intervention is important in the planning, timing and execution of vascular intervention.

Most busy vascular clinics now use a worksheet for a vascular examination.

Peripheral Vascular Worksheet

Important points to be covered in history are:

- History of food and drug allergies.
- Operations including cardiac or vascular intervention in the past.
- Obstetric history including miscarriages or deaths *in utero* (certain thrombophilias can cause these).
- Major illnesses in the past and their impact on the quality of life.

- Any history of serious infections, including multi-resistant organisms.
- History of deep venous thrombosis, pulmonary embolism, superficial thrombophlebitis, etc.
- Any cardiac history including angina, congestive heart failure, myocardial infarction, arrhythmias, nocturnal dyspnoea or dyspnoea on exertion.
- Any respiratory problems including chronic obstructive airways disease, asthma, lobectomy, occupational lung diseases, etc.
- Can this patient climb two flights of stairs without any effort? Can he blow out a matchstick at 15–20 cm?
- Diabetes including number of years, medications and the latest HbA1C levels.
- A history of stroke, transient ischaemic episodes, amaurosis fugax or peripheral neuropathy and a brief summary of treatment provided for these problems.
- Any history of venereal diseases or connective tissue diseases.
- Family history of diabetes, or cardiovascular morbidities including stroke, ischaemic heart disease, hypertension or clotting abnormalities.
- Personal history including alcohol, tobacco and recreational drug use.

Eliciting these points in history is important as they carry significant diagnostic and prognostic implications.

Complaints

Complaints	Rank	Severity	Descriptive comments
Pain			
Weakness			
Hot/cold			
Numb/sensitive			
Discolouration			
Swelling			
Ulceration			
Varicose veins			

Location

Location	Right/left	Medial/lateral	Dorsal/ventral
Toes/fingers			
Foot/hand			
Ankle/wrist			
Leg/forearm			
Knee/elbow			
Thigh/arm			
Hip/shoulder			
Back/neck			
Other			

Physical Examination

		Upper		Lower	
Extremities		Right	Left	Right	Left
Skin	Warm/cool				
	Atrophic/thickened				
	Cyanosis/mottling				
	Pallor/rubor				
	Capillary filling				
	Hair growth				
	Nails				
Oedema	Brawny/pitting/spongy				
	Degree				
	Extent				
Other findings	Subcutaneous atrophy/fibrosis				
	Ulceration/tissue loss				
	Discoloration/pigmentation				
	Erythema/cellulitis				
	Lymphangitis				

(Continued)

(*Continued*)

Extremities		Upper		Lower	
		Right	Left	Right	Left
Musculoskeletal	Symmetry/atrophy				
	Hypertrophy				
	Joint enlargement/swelling				
	Range of motion				
	Reflexes				
Neurology	Sensory				
	Motor				

Arterial Survey

	Right			Left		
	Pulse	Bruit	Aneurysm	Pulse	Bruit	Aneurysm
Carotid						
Subclavian						
Brachial						
Radial						
Ulnar						
Abdominal aorta						
Iliac						
Femoral						
Popliteal						
Posterior tibial						
Dorsalis pedis						

Venous survey N = normal, P = prominent/ tense, V = varicose, T = thrombosed		
	Right	Left
Great saphenous		
Lesser saphenous		
Anterolateral thigh		
Posteromedial thigh		
Anterior tibial		
Posterior tibial		
Posterior arch		
Perforators		
Intracutaneous venules		

Given the diffuse nature of vascular occlusive disease, it is essential to establish a pattern of examination so that few things are missed, if any. It is logical to examine the patient from head to toe. Start with the carotid pulse and keep the examination of foot pulses to the last. The equipment required for examination of a vascular patient is simple and consists of a stethoscope, a blood pressure cuff and a hand-held Doppler.

Examination of the Carotids

The patient is best examined in a semi-recumbent position with his head rested on a pillow. Thus, the sternocleidomastoid muscle is relaxed. The patient looks straight ahead. The carotid pulse can be palpated just lateral to the thyroid cartilage. The carotid bifurcation is variable and therefore one cannot assume that this pulse is due to the external, internal or the common carotid artery. One cannot assume either that the internal carotid artery is patent in a patient who has a palpable pulse as it could be the pulsation of the common carotid or the external carotid artery. It is essential to be gentle with palpation, especially in patients with history of amaurosis fugax, or transient ischaemic episodes. Rough palpation can dislodge plaque or precipitate bradycardia and vasovagal syncope. Gently supporting the head with the other hand during examination should evoke confidence in the patient. The carotid pulse should be followed

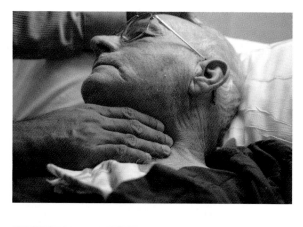

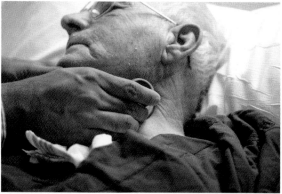

Figure 8.1.   Palpation and ascultation of the carotid artery.

down to the root of the neck to the ipsilateral sterno-clavicular joint. Compare the pulses on both aides. A very prominent pulse could be due to excessive tortuosity of the carotid artery or aneurymal disease and should be investigated further with a duplex scan.

Auscultation of the Carotid Artery

Ask the patient to breathe in and then breathe out. Ask him to hold his breath in expiration prior to placing the diaphragm of the stethoscope just lateral to the thyroid cartilage. A whooshing sound during systole could be due to plaque within the external carotid, the internal carotid or the common carotid artery. A bruit in presence of a stroke, a transient ischaemic episode or transient loss of vision in the ipsilateral eye should be viewed as significant and merits interrogation with duplex ultrasound. Approximately 3.5% of middle aged men and women have a carotid bruit and this incidence rises to 7% after the age of seventy. Less than 20% of carotid bruits are found to have any hemodynamic significance. Thus, carotid bruit in itself has very low specificity and should be considered significant only in the light of subsequent ultrasound findings and clinical correlation.

A soft systolo-diastolic bruit is likely to be due to increased flow through the superior thyroid artery as is seen with hyperthyroidism. An enlarged thyroid may be noted with other signs of hyperthyroidism such as exopthalmos.

It is difficult to differentiate a carotid bruit from a transmitted murmur from the heart due to aortic incompetence or aortic stenosis. A carotid bruit will not be heard at the root of the neck whilst a transmitted aortic murmur will be quite loud just above the sterno-clavicular joint and especially loud over the aortic area. Always ask the patient to hold his breath in expiration so that breath sounds or transmitted sounds do not mask a soft bruit.

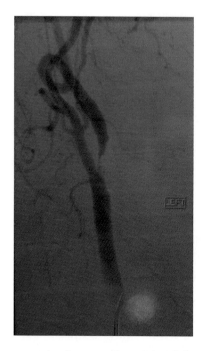

Figure 8.2. Smooth concentric plaque at the origin of the internal carotid artery causing a high-grade stenosis.

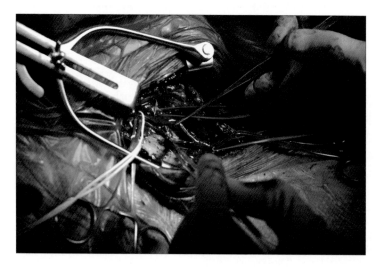

Figure 8.3. Carotid endarterectomy — high-grade calcific stenosis. Plaque elevated with a dissector.

Examination of the Upper Limb

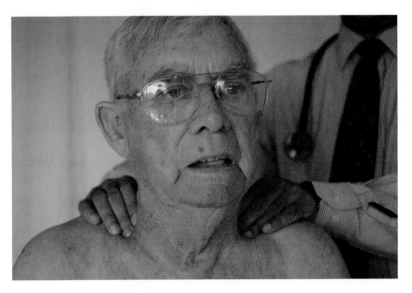

Figure 8.4. Palpation of the subclavian pulse in the supraclavicular fossa from behind.

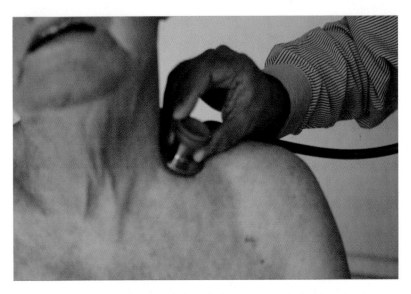

Figure 8.5. Auscultation of the subclavian artery in held expiration.

The subclavian pulses can be easily felt by sitting the semi-recumbent patient upright and turning him slightly so that you can stand behind him. Slide both hands over the bulk of the trapezius muscle to rest in the supraclavicular fossa on each side against the first rib. Moderate pressure exerted with the first three or four fingers of both hands will help appreciate the subclavian pulse on both sides simultaneously. Compare both pulses and then auscultate for a subclavian bruit in the supraclavicular fossa. Ask the patient to hold his breath in expiration during auscultation.

The axillary pulse is then palpated by rolling the artery against the humerus whilst supporting the flexed elbow with the other hand as seen in the picture. The axillary artery is readily palpable in its distal portion in the groove between the biceps and triceps muscles.

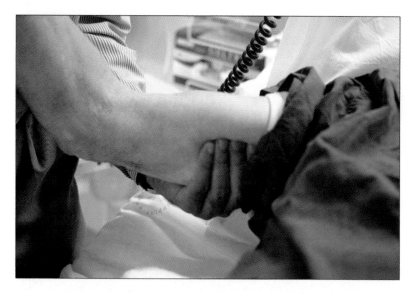

Figure 8.6.   Palpation of axillary pulse.

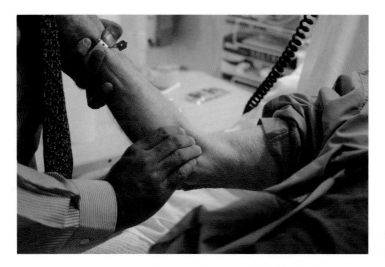

Figure 8.7. Palpation of brachial pulse medial to the biceps tendon.

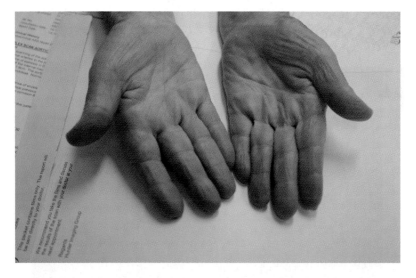

Figure 8.8. Cyanosis of fingertips in a patient with scleroderma — Raynaud's phenomenon.

The brachial artery is felt supporting the patient's flexed elbow so that the biceps tendon is relaxed. The brachial artery can be palpated just medial to the biceps tendon at the elbow crease.

The radial artery is readily palpable over the distal end of the radius just above the wrist. The ulnar pulse is difficult to feel as the artery is hidden behind the belly of flexor carpi ulnaris. It is however, still possible to feel the ulnar pulse with the wrist flexed and with some firm pressure. The ulnar artery is the dominant artery to the hand and its importance is frequently under-estimated. An Allen's test will help determine the dominant blood supply to the hand before attempting an invasive procedure such as insertion of a radial arterial line or catheterisation of the radial artery for a coronary angiogram. These procedures can be safely attempted as long as the ulnar contribution is intact.

Allen's Test

Blanching of fingers and palm with clenching and unclenching of fingers — while radial and ulnar arteries are compressed.

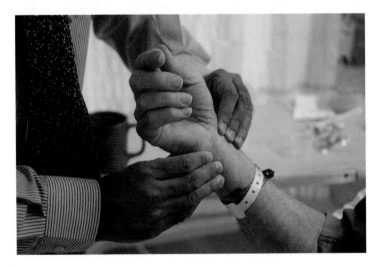

Figure 8.9. Simultaneous palpation of radial and ulnar pulses before proceeding with an Allen's test.

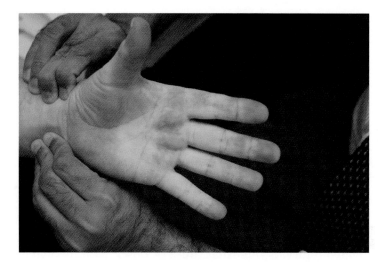

Figure 8.10.

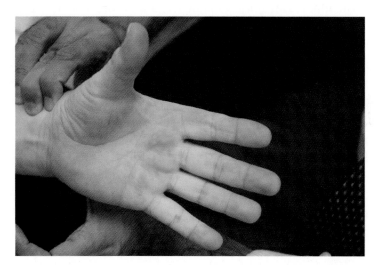

Figure 8.11.

Release of ulnar compression allows prompt return of colour to the hand indicating adequate flow via the ulnar artery. Similar test is performed to look for adequacy of flow from the radial component.

Special Tests to Diagnose Thoracic Outlet Syndrome

It is essential to check mobility at the shoulder, elbow and the wrist joint to rule out restricted joint mobility or contractures. There are three types of thoracic outlet syndrome: venous, neurological and arterial.

Neurogenic Thoracic Outlet Syndrome (TOS)

This is the commonest and accounts for 90% of thoracic outlet syndromes. Women in their third to fifth decades are affected. A single force trauma, such as a whiplash injury to the neck or a repetitive work related injury, is the usual cause of onset. Pain involving neck, shoulder, arm and hand in a descending order of frequency is the most common presenting symptom. Typically, there is tingling and numbness in the ulnar distribution of the hand and forearm. There may be recurrent headaches and patients usually cannot sleep on the affected side. Observe the seated patient's posture. Note any cervical or supraclavicular scars or deformities. A formal neurological examination for motor and sensory deficits in various muscle groups should be performed. Test for nerve entrapment at the carpal and cubital tunnel using a Phalen's and Tinel's test, respectively. Aggravation or induction of symptoms with a six-way motion of the neck while the affected limb is passively abducted to 90° suggests cervical disc disease.

Is there any tenderness over the brachial plexus on palpation? Reproduction of tingling and numbness or pain in the neck, shoulder or arm by focal compression over the anterior scalene muscle with fingertips denotes brachial plexus irritation. This is a characteristic finding of neurogenic TOS.

Adson's test

This test was in the past used to diagnose arterial TOS, but obliteration of the radial pulse occurs in 20% of the normal population with this manoeuvre. Therefore, it is now used only to reproduce irritation of the brachial plexus.

Contraction of the scalenus anterior is induced by having the patient turn the head away from the affected side and simultaneously taking a deep breath with the arm abducted to 90° and the elbow flexed to 90°. This manoeuvre may induce or aggravate sensory symptoms of neurogenic TOS due to simultaneous elevation of the first rib and contraction of the scalene muscles on that side. Bracing the shoulders backwards and downwards as in a military brace position narrows the thoracic outlet. Forcefully maintaining this position for 2–3 minutes will precipitate sensory symptoms.

The radial artery mainly supplies the deep palmar arch while the ulnar artery supplies the superficial palmar arch. These communicate freely with each other and maintain excel-

> **Kichu's thoughts . . .**
>
> The ulnar artery is the dominant artery of the hand and is often underestimated.

lent collateral supply to the hand. These anastomoses may be deficient or even absent at birth or due to diseases such as diabetes or scleroderma. Therefore, this test determines the contribution from the radial and ulnar arteries to the viability of the hand in the event one of these contributors fails.

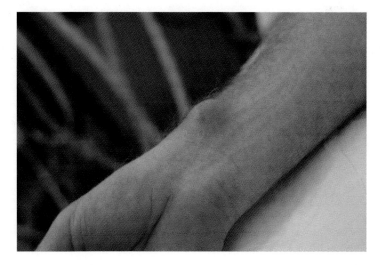

Figure 8.12. Pseudoaneurysm of radial artery following cardiac catheterisation before and during suergery.

The Upper Limb Tension Test

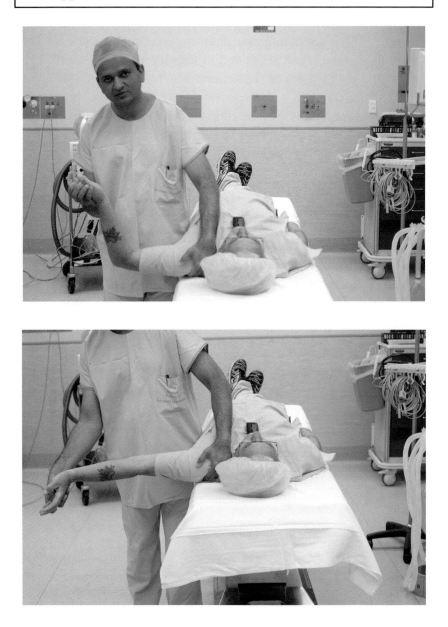

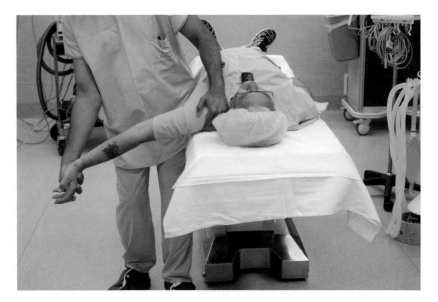

Figure 8.13. The upper limb tension test.

The patient lies supine. Stand on the side of the affected limb and gently support the shoulder with the palm of one hand. Now abduct the shoulder gently to 90° behind the coronal plane and externally rotate the shoulder. The elbow should then be brought to extension from 90° flexion in the horizontal plane with forearm in supination and the wrist extended. The result looks like a javelin thrower's action before release, the only difference is that it is done lying down. This test uses graduated tension on the brachial plexus until tightness, pain or worsening of symptoms occurs.

A double crush syndrome with co-existing cervical disk disease or nerve entrapment at the elbow or wrist makes those patients more susceptible to a neurogenic thoracic outlet syndrome.

Venous Thoracic Outlet Syndrome

There is extrinsic compression and repetitive trauma to the subclavian vein in the costoclavicular space. This narrow space is bounded by the anterior portion of the first rib forming the floor, the scalenus anterior

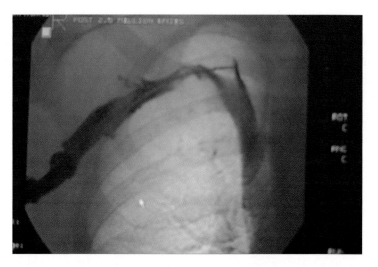

Figure 8.14. Compression of the subclavian vein demonstrated on venography — abrupt change in calibre of subclavian vein as it crosses over the first rib.

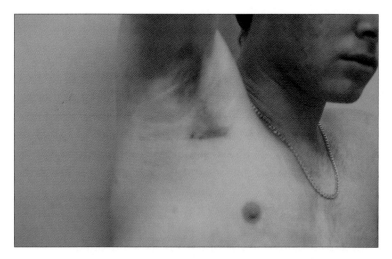

Figure 8.15. Transverse scar in the right axilla in the same patient after undergoing decompression of the subclavian by transaxillary resection of the first rib.

muscle forming the posterior border and the clavicle, the costoclavicular ligament and the subclavius muscle forming the anterior border. These patients are often young, athletic males with an overdeveloped upper body musculature due to physical conditioning or work.

Repeated compression of the subclavian vein leads to intimal fibrosis and thickening and an eventual occlusion of the axillosubclavian venous segment. These patients present with arm swelling aching, cyanosis, arm fatigue and venous distension over the affected limb as well as around the shoulder girdle. These symptoms and signs are exacerbated after exercising the affected limb. Large venous collaterals are seen over the deltopectoral region as well as the upper chest. The dominant arm is usually affected. Arm abduction narrows the costo-clavicular space causing venous distension of the affected extremity.

Arterial Thoracic Outlet Syndrome

This syndrome is less common than the neurogenic and venous types. These patients usually have an osseous abnormality of the first rib or an accessory rib or a myofascial band insinuating itself under-neath the subclavian artery. Most are young or middle aged men. Repetitive and forceful arm motion leads to focal compression of the subclavian artery leading to localised trauma. This leads to focal stenosis, ulceration with platelet thrombi or post-stenotic dilatation

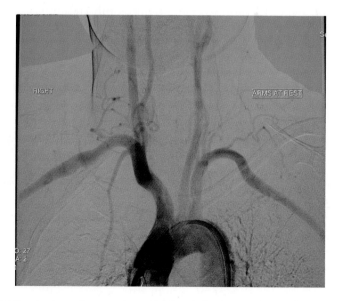

Figure 8.16.   Arch angiogram shows both subclavian arteries with arm resting by the sides.

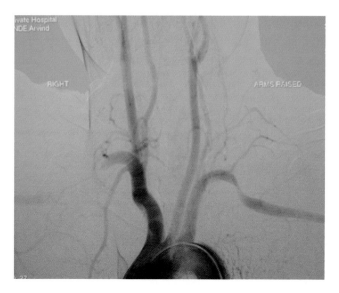

Figure 8.17. Arch aortogram showing occlusion of the right subclavian artery and stenosis of the left subclavian artery with arms raised overhead. The cause for constriction was bilateral cervical ribs.

and aneurysm formation. These patients present acutely with acute sub-clavian artery thrombosis threatening limb viability or persistent microembolization. A gradual occlusion of the subclavian artery is uncommon, but may present as muscle fatigue and cramps during exercise. Microembolisation leads to ischaemia and gangrene of the fingertips or a vaso-obstructive Raynaud's. An abnormal unilateral Allen's test indicates microembolisation rather than any other systemic cause.

Blood pressure is taken from both arms after palpation of pulses and may be lower on the affected side due to stenosis of the subclavian artery. The subclavian artery on the affected side may be unduly prominent due to it being elevated over the underlying osseous or myofascial sling. A post-stenotic dilatation or aneurysm of the subclavian artery may result in a prominent pulse. Abduction at the shoulder to 90° with the elbow flexed to 90° and externally rotated may obliterate the radial pulse (EAST test) and repeated clasping and unclasping of fingers in this position will quickly lead to tingling numbness and ischaemic pain in the affected limb. Auscultation for a subclavian bruit should be performed in a neutral and EAST position.

Examination of the Abdomen

Inspection and palpation of the abdomen should be performed as is standard in any clinical examination. On inspection, a prominent abdominal pulsation may indicate an abdominal aortic aneurysm or an ectatic tortuous abdominal aorta. Abdominal scars may indicate previous vascular surgery or other abdominal surgery. Gentle palpation around a pulsatile abdominal lump should give a rough idea about the size of the aneurysm. If one is able to feel the upper border of the aneurysm and insinuate fingers between the costal margin and the aneurysm, then it is likely that this aneurysm is infrarenal. Approximately 95% of abdominal aortic aneurysms are infrarenal. Nearly 10% of abdominal aortic aneurysms are associated with popliteal artery aneurysms. On the other hand, 40% of patients with bilateral popliteal aneurysms have an abdominal aortic aneurysm. Therefore, a high index of suspicion should be maintained about the co-existence of abdominal and popliteal aneurysmal disease. Rarely enlarged para-aortic lymph nodes can mimic an abdominal aortic aneurysm. On

> **Kichu's thoughts . . .**
>
> A tender aortic aneurysm must be referred for urgent surgical evaluation.

palpation of an abdominal aortic aneurysm along its lateral borders simultaneously with both index fingers aligned parallel to the long axis of the aneurysm, there will be an upward and outward movement of the fingers. This is an expansible impulse whereas with a para-aortic lymph node mass, only an upward impulse (non-expansile) will be transmitted. A bruit may be auscultated over an abdominal aortic aneurysm due to turbulence in the sac. A duplex scan will help with accurate sizing of the anteroposterior diameter of the aneurysm sac. This is the single most important determinant of the risk of rupture.

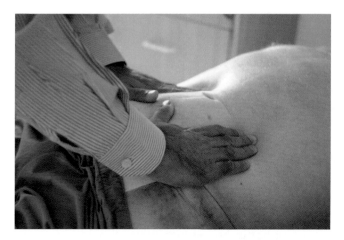

Figure 8.18. Palpation of abdominal aortic aneurysm — estimation of approximate diameter. Fingers move upwards and outwards indicating an expansile impulse.

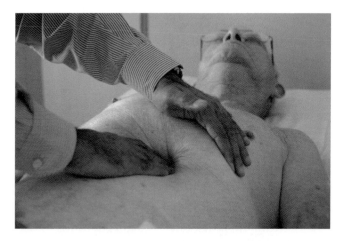

Figure 8.19. Insinuation of fingers between the costal margin and the upper limit of the aneurysm indicates an infrarenal aneurysm.

Epigastric bruit in presence of resistant hypertension should raise the suspicion of renal artery stenosis. Patients with an epigastric bruit, significant weight loss and abdominal pain on ingestion of food may have superior mesenteric artery stenosis with or without a stenosis at the origin of the celiac axis. A duplex ultrasound examination is helpful in diagnosis of mesenteric ischaemia as well as renovascular hypertension. Many asymptomatic patients may have an epigastric bruit; not much significance can then be attached to this finding.

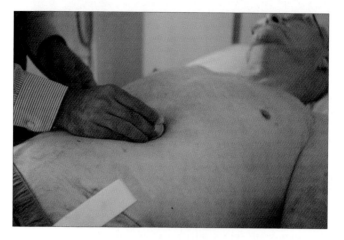

Figure 8.20. Ascultation of the bruit.

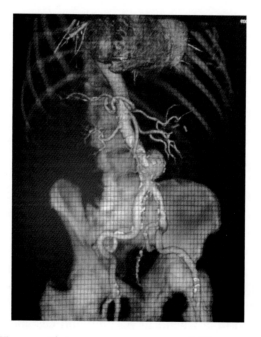

Figure 8.21. CT scan with intravenous contrast and 3D reconstruction shows a large aneurysm at the aortic bifurcation.

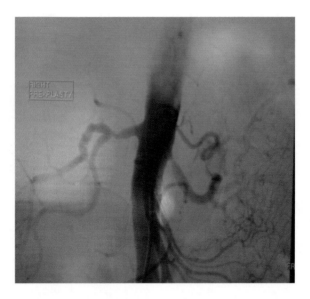

Figure 8.22. Angiogram shows bilateral renal artery stenosis in a young patient with hypertension and epigastric bruit.

Very rarely, young asthenic females with weight loss and abdominal pain after eating may present with an epigastric bruit only during expiration. This is due to the compression of the celiac axis by the median arcuate ligament connecting the two diaphragmatic crura as the abdominal viscera ascends during expiration.

Examination of the Lower Limbs

Inspection of lower limbs: A gross inspection will reveal the presence of any hip or knee contractures. Does the patient prefer to place the affected extremity in a dependent position?

Is there a fungal infection of the nails leading to deformity and brittle nails? Is there fungal infection or bacterial infection in the web spaces as is common with diabetic foot? Is there any loss of hair over the affected extremity? Is the skin pale atrophic and shiny? If the affected foot is bright red in a dependent position and becomes pale on elevation, this denotes vasomotor paralysis due to advanced ischaemia.

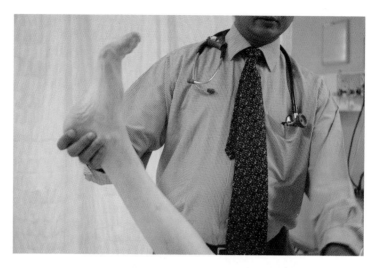

Figure 8.23. Elevation of an ischaemic leg with resultant pallor and guttering of veins.

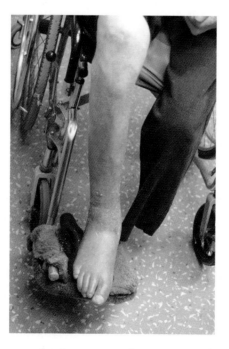

Figure 8.24. The same leg becomes erythematous on dependency. Have you noticed that the left leg has been amputated previously?

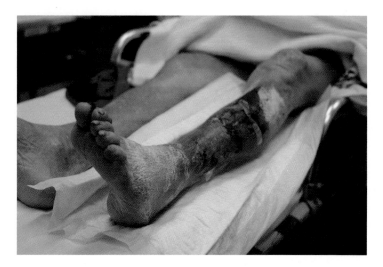

Figure 8.25.   Dead insensate leg with fixed mottling.

If the skin over the foot or lower leg is mottled, then this may indicate advanced ischaemia. If pressure fails to displace the mottling, this indicates advanced and probably irreversible ischaemia. Fixed mottling is a poor prognostic sign, especially in association with sensorimotor paralysis and these limbs cannot be salvaged.

Measure the girth of the thighs and calves at their maximum bulk. Patients with chronic ischaemia will have some loss of muscle bulk in the affected extremity. Any obvious ankle or foot deformity may indicate a disorganised foot in a diabetic patient. This is called a Charcot's foot. An imbalance between the long flexors and extensors due to loss of the small intrinsic muscles may lead to clawing of toes or hammer toes. A hallux valgus with an infected or ulcerated bunion over the ball of the first toe in an elderly female may be the first sign of underlying ischaemia.

Asking the patient to perform an aerial cycle whilst supine will test the mobility of the hip and knee joints and the power and flexibility of the muscles that move these joints. Active flexion and extension at the ankle will be affected if there is any sensory or motor paralysis.

Palpation of Arterial Pulses

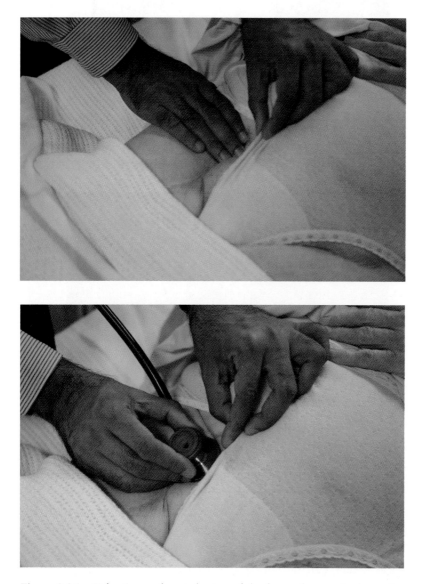

Figure 8.26.   Palpation and auscultation of the femoral artery in the groin.

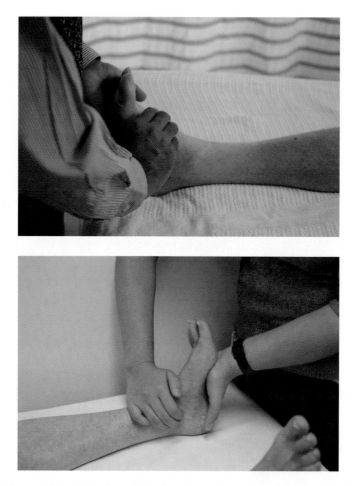

Figure 8.27. Palpation of the dorsalis pedis and the posterior tibial pulse.

It is good practice to feel pulses in the asymptomatic limb and compare with the affected side. Slight abduction and external rotation at the hip is helpful in palpation of the femoral pulse in an obese patient. The femoral pulse is sought at finger's breadth lateral and below the pubic tubercle at the mid-inguinal point. Frequently, the femoral artery can be rolled against the superior pubic ramus as a thickened calcified structure in the elderly and in diabetic patients.

This should be followed by auscultation at this point for a bruit, if a thrill is not obvious. A bruit or a thrill in the groin indicates turbulent blood flow due to calcific plaque upstream. This is a common finding in aortoiliac occlusive disease.

The popliteal pulse is felt with the patient supine and relaxed. The knee joint is flexed to 15–20° in order to relax the dense, fibrous, overlying popliteal fascia. Both thumbs are placed anteriorly on the tibial tuberosity and the fingers are wrapped around the calf just below the

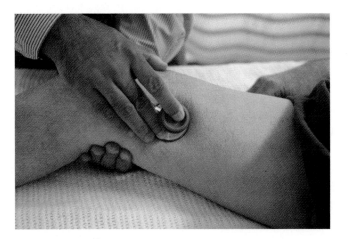

Figure 8.28.   Auscultation at the adductor hiatus. A bruit indicates plaque in the common femoral or the proximal superficial artery.

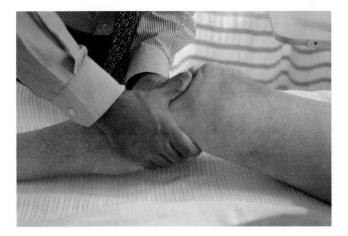

Figure 8.29.   The popliteal pulse is sought over the back of the tibial plateau by partly flexing the knee and thus relaxing the popliteal fascial envelope.

knee crease. The popliteal pulse is felt with gradually increasing pressure over the posterior aspect of the tibia. A prominent popliteal pulse usually denotes popliteal aneurysmal disease or ectasia. Auscultation over the adductor hiatus can demonstrate a bruit, especially if there is a calcific lesion in the common femoral or the superficial femoral artery.

The posterior tibial pulse is felt in the hollow behind the medial malleolus. Gently support the patient's foot on the plantar surface so that the foot is kept neutral. The dorsalis pedis pulse is absent in approximately 10% of the population. This artery is felt just lateral to the tendon of the extensor hallucis longus in the groove between the first and second metatarsal bones. The foot should be gently supported on the plantar surface during palpation.

Passive flexion and extension at the hip, knee and ankle joint is essential to rule out contractures. Patients with rest-pain over a long duration tend to hold their leg in a semi-flexed dependent position and it is not uncommon to find knee contracture in these patients. A contracture of the knee joint effectively precludes a salvage operation and creates problems with below-knee amputations.

Role of Hand-held Doppler and Photoplethysmography in Assessing Vascular Reserve

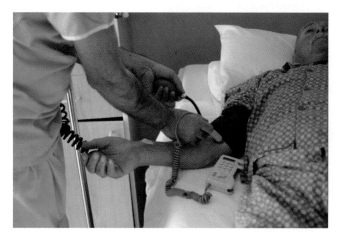

Figure 8.30.   Measurement of systolic pressure in the brachial artery for assessment of the ankle-brachial pressure index.

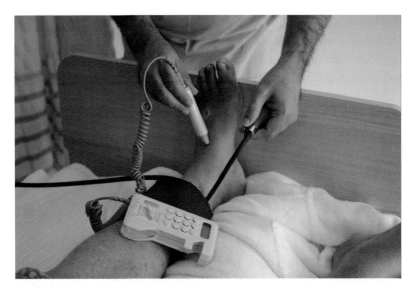

Figure 8.31.   Measurement of systolic pressure in the dorsalis pedis with a 10 MHz Doppler probe.

A hand-held continous-wave Doppler probe with a frequency of 8–10 MHz is used for measuring the ankle-brachial pressure index. For best results, the probe should be angled at 45–60° to the long axis of the vessel. A blood pressure cuff should ideally have a width of 20 percent more than the diameter of the extremity for accurate measurement of the systolic blood pressure. A blood pressure cuff is first applied around the arm and a triphasic waveform is heard once the Doppler probe is placed over the brachial artery just medial to the bicipital tendon at the elbow crease with the elbow relaxed and flexed to 90°. A triphasic signal sounds like a whiplash and the probe is angled and positioned to hear the best signal. Some ultrasound gel is applied to the tip of the probe prior to placement in order to allow good coupling to the underlying soft tissue. Without the coupling gel, signals will not be heard due to acoustic impedance from the tissue–air interface. Keeping the probe steady, the blood pressure cuff is gradually inflated until the Doppler signals disappear. Inflate the cuff to 20 mmHg above this level and then gradually deflate the cuff until the Doppler signal begins to return. This is the brachial occlusive systolic pressure. An appropriate blood pressure cuff is then applied just above the ankle and Doppler signals are again sought over the dorsalis pedis and the posterior tibial pulses at the ankle. The systolic occlusive pressures are recorded. The higher systolic pressure out of the two pulses interrogated at the ankle is used for calculating the ankle brachial index. For example, if the systolic occlusive pressure over the posterior tibial artery is higher than that over the dorsalis pedis, then the posterior tibial pressure should be divided by the brachial systolic occlusive pressure to calculate the ankle brachial pressure index. If the radial pulses are unequal, then compare bilateral brachial pressures and use the higher out of the two for the calculation. The left subclavian artery is six times more likely to be affected by significant occlusive plaque at its origin than the right side.

An ankle-brachial index of 1.1 to 0.9 is normal. An index below 0.9 up to 0.6 denotes reasonable vascular reserve and is usually found in mild claudicants. An index below 0.6 denotes a greatly diminished vascular reserve and is found in short distance claudicants. An index below 0.35 indicates critical ischaemia requiring prompt intervention and is usually found in patients with multilevel occlusive disease or severe calf vessel disease with tissue loss or gangrene.

An ankle-brachial index of more than 1.2 is to be discarded as it usually means that the calf arteries are hard to compress such as in diabetes or patients with scleroderma or end-stage renal failure. These patients have calf vessels that are very hard to compress.

In this group of patients, a photoplethysmography probe is secured over the pulp of the big toe or the second toe. An appropriately sized pneumatic cuff is wrapped around the toe. Infrared waves transmitted by the probe are reflected back from the subdermal capillary plexus with minimal attenuation. Each waveform corresponds to inflow and egress of blood from the pulp space. Inflate the pneumatic cuff until the waveform is obliterated on the display. An absolute toe pressure of less than 30 mmHg indicates severe vascular insufficiency and urgent vascular intervention is required. Toe pressures between 30 and 60 mmHg are labelled as borderline ischaemia

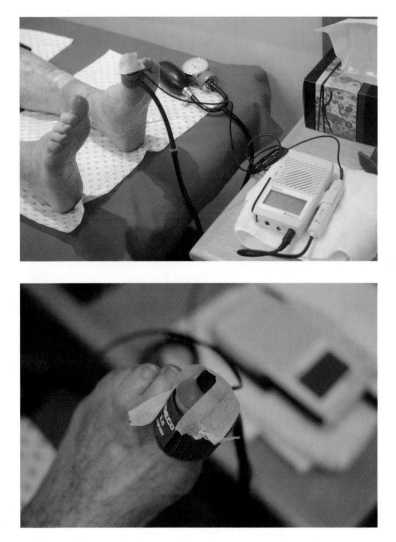

Figure 8.32.   Toe occlusive pressure measures the perfusion pressure in the digital arteries with a photoplethysmography probe and a miniature blood pressure cuff.

and these patients require careful surveillance and wound management. Absolute toe pressures above 60 mmHg denote that an ulcer or area of tissue loss may have good healing potential if other underlying causes, such as inappropriate pressure or infection, are removed.

The Painful Limb

Chronic arterial insufficiency can have a serious impact on the quality of life or lead to eventual disability and death if left untreated.

Patients with chronic arterial insufficiency suffer from:

• Claudication
• Rest pain

Claudication is a cramping pain consistently reproduced in a muscle group by the same degree of exercise and completely relieved by a minute or so of rest.

Though the commonest affected sites are the calves, buttocks, thighs or even feet can be affected depending on the level and extent of arterial occlusion.

Patients with a predominantly aortoiliac occlusion or stenosis complain of cramping in the buttocks and upper thighs and sometimes in the calves. In men, there may be additional vasculogenic impotence. Impotence associated with aortoiliac occlusive disease and buttock and thigh claudication is called Leriche's syndrome. Femoropopliteal occlusive disease usually leads to calf claudication. High-grade stenosis of the common femoral artery can lead to extremely short distance claudication as the blood flow to the profunda femoris and the superficial femoral artery is affected. Femoropopliteal occlusive disease and aortoiliac stenosis, classically occurs in smokers. Calf claudication at short distances can be a result of occlusive lesions in the calf arteries; these lesions are predominantly seen in patient with diabetes.

Foot claudication is very rare and is usually a precursor to ischaemic rest pain. It only occurs with advanced degrees of arterial insufficiency. It has been classically described in thromboangiitis obliterans as there is a typically a diffuse and distal distribution of occlusive lesions. These patients complain of a gnawing pain or cramps in the forefoot.

Conditions Mimicking Calf Claudication

Nocturnal cramps in calves in older patients are not due to ischaemia, but occur most probably due to an exaggerated neuromuscular

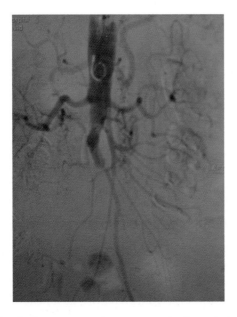

Figure 8.33. Abdominal aortogram shows a completely occluded abdominal aorta just below the renal arteries in a patient with aortoiliac occlusive disease. This patient suffered from short distance claudication mainly in the buttocks and thighs.

response to stretch. These respond very well to calcium and magnesium supplements, despite there being no documented deficiency.

Athletes or runners can complain of tightness in calves precipitated by exercise. This group has overdeveloped calf musculature. In a chronic compartment syndrome, pain comes on after considerable exercise and then subsides very slowly with rest. Increased blood flow leads to muscle swelling and impaired venous outflow within an unyielding fascial envelope, leading to pain, tightness in calf, absent foot pulses and numbness in the foot.

Functional popliteal entrapment is due to hypertrophic gastrocnemius and soleus muscles leading to intermittent compression of the popliteal artery, especially during prolonged exercise leading to muscle ischaemia, swelling and then progression towards a chronic compartment syndrome. These patients have palpable pulses at rest and abnormalities are detected on a stress treadmill test or with compartment pressures only after prolonged exercise. Patients with overdeveloped calf muscles can occlude their popliteal arteries with active plantar flexion and with prolonged exercise, as seen quite easily on arterial duplex combined with stress treadmill pressure indices.

Venous claudication due to unresolved deep venous obstruction following ileofemoral or femoropopliteal deep venous thrombosis, can cause thigh and/or calf claudication. As recanalization has not occurred in these patients, there is engorgement of superficial and deep venous channels causing a tight or bursting sensation. There are accompanying signs of venous congestion, dermatitis, pigmentation and edema. This sensation does not abate quickly after cessation of exercise but relief is speeded by leg elevation.

Nerve root compression due to a herniated disc can cause a sharp cutting or burning pain which radiates down the leg. This pain starts variably after or with exercise and is relieved only by adjusting position or posture, or leaning against something. This pain takes more time to disappear than true vascular claudication. There is a history of back problems and a MRI or CT of the lumbosacral spine can lead to the diagnosis. These patients have a normal arterial duplex and a stress treadmill test does not lead to reduction in the ankle-brachial pressure indices.

Osteoarthritis of the knee joint can imitate claudication as well. These patients have crepitus over the knee joint during passive flexion and extension. These patients have a variable amount of pain during walking, as well as some pain or discomfort at night when worn out joint surfaces rub against each other in absence of surrounding muscle spasm.

Conditions Mimicking Buttock and Thigh Claudication

Osteoarthritis of the hip joint can cause pain in the hip thighs and buttocks. There is usually a deep-seated ache and discomfort after a variable degree of exercise. Changes in weather conditions and physical activity impact the severity of pain. This pain or discomfort may or may not be quickly relieved with rest but there is a definite improvement in symptoms once weight is taken off the legs.

Neurospinal compression (spinal claudication) is caused by narrowing of the lumbar spinal canal due to osteophytes. This causes pain or discomfort and weakness in the hips, thighs and buttocks.

However, the onset is variable and can occur not only with walking, but even with prolonged standing, lifting heavy weights or violent coughing. These patients usually have to sit down and sometimes stoop forwards (lumbar flexion), in order to gain relief. These patients usually have a history of backache.

Conditions Mimicking Foot Claudication

Foot claudication in itself is a very rare condition. Therefore, arthritic or inflammatory conditions of the foot must be excluded before entertaining this diagnosis. Sharp severe pain and numbness in the foot with prolonged standing or walking with associated clinical signs, including tenderness over joints or synovial thickening, should be followed up with an MRI or foot X-ray and a bone scan.

Rest Pain

This is typically a diffuse and severe nocturnal pain mostly involving the forefoot. It is the cry of dying nerves and may, therefore, not be adequately relieved even with large doses of narcotics. These patients cannot lie horizontal and tend to sleep in a chair or hang their foot out of the bed.

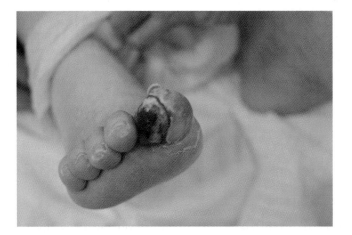

Figure 8.34. POUCH dependent (rest pain, dependant oedema, ulceration, colour changes and hyperaesthesia) denote critical ischaemia and impending loss of limb.

The pulses in the affected limb are diminished or absent. The foot pulses are invariably impalpable. With the patient supine, raising the foot to 30° above the horizontal leads to cadaveric pallor over the dorsum, the pulp spaces of the toes and the plantar aspect of the foot, along with guttering of superficial veins over the dorsum of the foot.

If the foot is then placed in a dependent position, there is rubor over the dorsum and the plantar surface of the foot. There is slow refilling of the guttered veins as compared to the relatively unaffected contralateral limb. This rubor is due to a gravity-dependent inrush of blood in to a chronically-dilated vascular bed. These patients usually have atrophy of the calf muscles along with loss of hair over the dorsum of the foot. There may be associated thickening and deformity of toe nails due to fungal infection and loss of nourishment to the nail bed. In a horizontal position, the normal time for the return of capillary blush over digits is less than two seconds. In critical ischaemia, this capillary refill time exceeds two seconds (the time required to say "capillary refill").

Differential for Rest Pain

Early stages of diabetic neuropathy can be mistaken for rest pain. This pain is due to neuritis with a symmetrical stocking-like distribution. However, these patients may also have diminished foot pulses and dependent rubor and trophic skin changes due to the accompanying destruction of sympathetic nerves. This picture may also be seen in other types of peripheral neuritis.

Degenerative or inflammatory arthritis in the foot such as gout can mimic rest pain, but this pain is exacerbated by putting weight on the foot and walking. This metatarsalgia is variable and at times, it may be absent for a few days. Foot pulses are invariably present. There may be associated pin point tenderness over the small bones or joints in the foot.

Morton's metatarsalgia

Repeated trauma to the plantar digital nerves due to a milking action between metatarsal heads may lead to painful traumatic neuromas. These can mimic rest pain in the presence of foot pulses.

Reflex sympathetic dystrophy can cause as much pain and distress as rest pain and can be either as the result of an incomplete nerve injury or relatively minor trauma to the affected limb. The pain is of a burning nature with an irregular and diffuse distribution. It is out of proportion to the physical signs. This pain is not only in the forefoot, but usually affects the entire limb up to or above the level of the knee. The signs of autonomic imbalance are marked. The limb displays marked vasomotor changes in response to physical stress or emotions. The affected limb may initially be warm and dry but later becomes cool mottled and cyanotic. This pain is relieved effectively with a sympathetic block. Peripheral pulses are usually present despite cyanosis and mottling.

Patients with any of the above conditions may have absent or attenuated peripheral pulses and in these patients, toe occlusion pressure with a photoplethysmography probe is useful in differentiating critical ischaemia from non-vascular causes.

Acute Ischaemia

Embolism causes acute ischaemia. Arterial thrombosis occurs with pre-existing arterial disease and these patients mostly have a pre-existing history of claudication. With acute embolism, there is usually an underlying cause such as atrial fibrillation, recent history of myocardial infarction, aortic or popliteal aneurysm, ventricular aneurysm or patent foramen ovale. These causes may not be evident in the initial evaluation. In young patients, thrombophilia should be kept in mind.

The classic signs of advanced acute ischaemia or acute on chronic ischaemia are pain, pallor, pulseless, paraesthesia, paralysis and perishing cold.

Sensorimotor paralysis indicates an advanced irreversible ischaemia and mandates prompt intervention if life and limb are to be saved.

To detect early motor weakness, it is essential to test the intrinsic muscles of the foot rather than the long flexors and extensors as these are affected much later. Capillary refill is markedly delayed and peripheral pulses are absent.

The pain in acute embolism is severe and diffuse. It begins suddenly and most patients describe a sensation of being struck in the leg by a severe shocking pain along with weakness. These symptoms may not be present in arterial thrombosis where the patient becomes aware that his/her pre-existing claudication has worsened and is now replaced by unremitting rest pain.

Embolic episodes can resolve spontaneously especially in patients who are heparinised promptly and many of these patients may notice an immediate improvement in their pain and weakness as the initial vasospasm subsides and the embolic load breaks up restoring flow in the major vessels and collateral branches.

With arterial thrombosis, the initial ischaemic insult may be relieved as vasospasm subsides and pre-existing collateral channels are recruited, but claudication may still remain.

Overview of Vascular Pathologies Affecting Lower Arteries

Diabetic Foot

Patients with diabetes suffer from accelerated atherosclerosis and this reflects in the involvement of medium and small sized arteries. Diabetic smokers can have aortoiliac, femoropopliteal or calf vessel occlusive disease in varying combination. The common factor is the presence of diffuse calcification of the aortoiliac, femoropopliteal and calf arteries. This calcification renders these arteries almost incompressible. Measurement of ankle-brachial pressure indices in these patients is therefore not useful.

These patients have a predominant involvement of the motor and sensory nerves in their lower limbs. As there is also a concomitant involvement of the sympathetic nerves, these patients have dry scaly lichenified skin with warmth and erythema. Initially, there is neuropathic pain but eventually these patients progress to insensate feet. As the proprioceptive receptors in the foot and ankle joint are also affected, these patients can load certain areas of their feet and this leads to degeneration and collapse of some of the small joints. As the intrinsic muscles in the foot are affected, the balance between

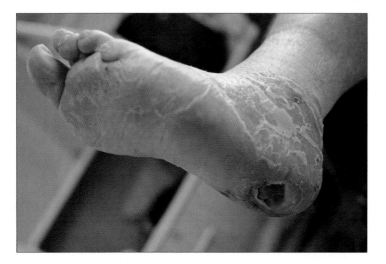

Figure 8.35.   Neuropathic diabetic foot syndrome.

the long flexors and extensors is affected, leading to a flat foot or a high arched foot, hammer toes or swan neck deformity of the toes, a valgus or varus deformity at the ankle as well as at the meta-tarsophalangeal joints.

The end result is an insensate foot with a grossly disorganised bony architecture called a Charcot's foot. There is ulceration over bony pressure points especially over the metatarsal heads, commonly the first and second. Eventually osteomyelitis and deep space infection of the plantar surface sets in. Foot pulses, are, however, still present.

Though the popliteal pulse may be present, foot pulses are absent. Ulcers are predominantly on the tips of toes and there is associated pain.

There is a predominant involvement of the calf arteries (the posterior and anterior tibial arteries, as well as the peroneal artery). The medial and lateral plantar arteries, as well as the dorsalis pedis arteries, may also be variably involved. The end result is a diffuse occlusive pattern involving the calf arteries and the foot vessels. These patients may have rest pain if peripheral nerves are still unaffected. As the vessels in the calf and foot are heavily calcified,

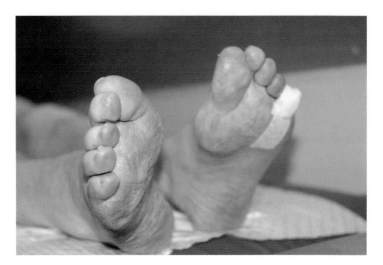

Figure 8.36.   Ischaemic diabetic foot syndrome.

the digital arteries are relatively unaffected. Therefore, a toe occlusion pressure with a photoplethysmography probe and a miniature
blood pressure cuff wrapped around the first or second toe is most
useful in assessing vascular reserve. These patients may have damaged sympathetic nerves; therefore, a dependent foot will appear
erythematous, well-perfused and warm to touch. However, elevat-
ing the leg (Buerger's test) will drain the foot of blood and render
it white.

Neuroischaemic diabetic foot

This is the most common presentation of a diabetic foot. There is neuropathy as well as occlusive disease of the calf vessels and vessels in the
foot. These patients may present with an ischaemic ulcer on the toes
or with a trophic ulcer over the pressure-bearing areas of the foot, such
as the first or second meta-tarsophalangeal joints on the plantar aspect.
Pain is absent or reduced due to associated neuropathy. Lack of sympathetic nerve supply causes rubor and warmth in the dependent lower
limb. An associated infection may contribute to the warmth. A
Buerger's test is strongly positive. Associated nerve damage may result

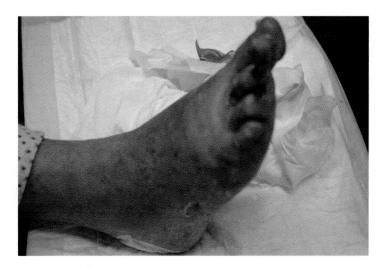

in various deformities and degenerative changes, including a Charcot's foot. A toe occlusion pressure is extremely useful in assessing vascular reserve in these patients.

Aorto-iliac Occlusive Disease

There are three distinct patterns of infrarenal vascular occlusive disease. An overlap and presence of two or all three occlusive patterns together is called a multilevel occlusive disease and this causes critical lower limb ischaemia.

Aortoiliac occlusive disease in itself usually presents as buttock and thigh claudication relieved by rest. Involvement of the internal iliac and the common iliac arteries can result in vasculogenic impotence in men. A harsh bruit on auscultation and a thrill on palpating the femoral arteries due to turbulence in the iliac arteries is common. The femoral pulses may be weak or unequal. At times, some of this plaque can disrupt and the resulting athero-embolism can result in occlusion of digital or metatarsal arteries with a blue or gangrenous toe in presence of good foot pulses.

Patients with aortoiliac occlusive disease are usually heavy smokers.

Femoropopliteal occlusive disease afflicts smokers and results in crippling short distance calf claudication if the compensation by genicular collaterals is inadequate. These patients have strong femoral pulses if there is no coexisting aortoiliac occlusive disease. The popliteal pulse and foot pulses are absent. There is loss of hair on the shin and foot with shiny atrophic skin in advanced ischaemia. The superficial femoral artery is usually occluded. The claudication symptoms are usually more severe if the common femoral artery or the profunda femoris are affected. The profunda femoris is rarely stenosed except at its origin due to plaque in the common femoral artery. The profunda femoris is very rarely affected in its mid-portion or distally and then only in diabetics or patients with scleroderma.

Tibioperoneal occlusive affects the calf arteries and is typically seen in diabetics, patients with connective tissue diseases or vasculitis (Buerger's disease) or renal failure. Some elderly patients may also have this disease. The peroneal artery is generally spared, but the anterior tibial and posterior tibial are affected. Even if the peroneal artery is unaffected, its terminal branches, the anterior and posterior perimalleolar tibial branches may be occluded so that the critical run-off into the dorsalis pedis or posterior tibial is affected, leading to critical ischaemia. These patients have a palpable popliteal pulse but absent foot pulses. Calf claudication is the presenting symptom until critical ischaemia sets in.

Popliteal Entrapment Syndrome

This condition results from a developmental anomaly wherein the popliteal artery passes medial to and beneath the medial head of the gastrocnemius muscle or through the belly of this muscle. Rarely, the popliteus muscle may trap the popliteal artery to the posterior surface of the tibia, causing compression. Very rarely may a hypertrophied medial and lateral gastrocnemius muscle or the soleus-plantaris muscle complex in an athletic individual cause functional compression. Repetitive compression of the popliteal artery by the medial head of gastrocnemius eventually leads to adventitial thickening, then medial thickening and fragmentation and, finally, damage to the endothelium. At first, there is narrowing of the artery. This is followed by fixed narrowing in the non-reversible stage, finally leading to thrombosis of a short segment of the popliteal artery. Claudication in a young man or woman should raise suspicion. It occurs more frequently in men. Symptoms range from mild claudication with exercise or vigorous walking through to short distance claudication or rest pain with critical ischaemia. Foot pulses readily palpable with the foot in a neutral position are obliterated with passive dorsiflexion of the foot or on active plantar flexion. This diagnosis is further reinforced by duplex ultrasound and a confirmatory diagnosis is reached with an angiogram with and without resisted plantar flexion. This angiogram may show marked medial deviation of the popliteal artery, segmental occlusion or post-stenotic dilatation. A magnetic resonance angiogram may actually show the anatomic structure causing compression of the artery.

Adventitial cystic disease of the popliteal artery

This rare condition is another important differential diagnosis in young patients with calf claudication. This condition is seen predominantly in males in their fourth and fifth decades. There is sudden onset of claudication at a short distance due to compression of the popliteal artery by a mucoid cyst arising in the adventitia. Duplex examination shows a boundary between the cyst contents and the vessel lumen as a fine bright line that pulsates in real time. MRI scan usually confirms the diagnosis.

Vasculitis

One of the most prominent conditions in this group of patients is thromboangiitis obliterans.

Thromboangiitis obliterans

This is a segmental inflammatory disease affecting the small and medium sized arteries and veins in the upper and lower limbs.

These patients are heavy users of tobacco, though occasionally, it has also been associated with the use of marijuana. This condition is more prevalent in the Middle East and the Indian subcontinent than Europe or North America. An important difference from other types of vasculitis is the absence in the rise in the ESR, CRP, immune complexes, ANA, RA factor and complement levels. Rarely, cerebral, coronary, mesenteric or renal vessels can be involved.

These patients are typically young males before the age of 45 years who are heavy smokers. They may present with claudication in the feet or ischaemic ulceration. These patients may show clinical evidence of upper limb involvement such as an absent radial or ulnar pulse or an abnormal Allen's test. They commonly exhibit Raynaud's phenomenon in the upper and lower limbs. Migratory superficial thrombophlebitis is another typical feature in the active phase of the disease. TAO is a diagnosis of exclusion. Laboratory tests to document the distal nature of the disease include duplex scans, pulse volume recording and laboratory tests to exclude autoimmune and hypercoagulable states. A cardiac echo is useful to exclude a proximal source of emboli. Angiography helps exclude a proximal embolic source such as a plaque, but also reveals typical diagnostic features. Angiography shows involvement of small and medium sized arteries with a segmental distribution. Typical corkscrew collaterals are seen.

Examination of the Venous System

Varicose veins

These are large superficial veins that become very prominent and stand out like cords when the patient stands up and therefore should be examined standing up.

Primary varicose veins occur in familial clusters and are due to congenital aplasia or hypoplasia of valves in superficial veins along with dilatation of valve rings due to lack of supporting connective tissue. These may be further exacerbated by occupational demands such as standing up for prolonged periods of time or due to the hormonal influences as well as and IVC and iliac vein compression in pregnancy. Varicose veins usually regress after pregnancy. Large pelvic or abdominal tumours may cause pressure effects and lead to varicose veins.

Secondary varicose veins are due to destruction of valves in the deep veins and perforators secondary to deep venous thrombosis and subsequent recanalization. Thus, there is direct transmission of pressure from an incompetent deep venous system via incompetents perforators to the superficial venous system. A past history of trauma, fracture or an orthopaedic procedure may point towards an episode of DVT.

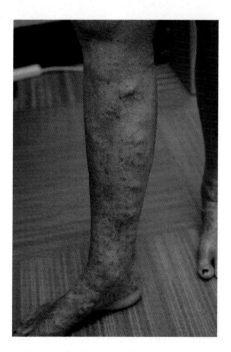

Figure 8.37. Varicosities in the long saphenous territory. Note pigmentation around the ankle due to distal venous pigmentation.

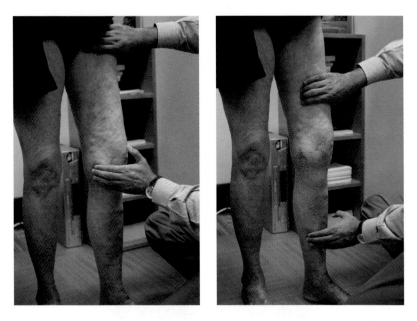

Figure 8.38.   Palpation for an impulse at the saphenofemoral junction followed by a tap on prominent varicosities below the knee.

There are two distinct territories. The long saphenous territory starts from the groin and extends all the way down to the medial malleolus along the course of the long saphenous vein. The antero-lateral vein of the thigh and the posteromedial vein of the thigh are the major tributaries of the long saphenous vein in thigh and these may have varicosities associated with them. Below the knee, there may be varicosities associated with the anterolateral vein of calf or the posterior arch vein. Varicosities associated with the long saphen-ous territory are almost never over the lateral part or posterolateral aspect of the calf. The short saphenous vein courses posteriorly from the popliteal fossa to the lateral malleolus and therefore varicosities associated with this vein are in the posterior posterolateral and lat-eral aspect of the calf.

Thus, a quick determination of the long saphenous and short saphenous territory will determine whether there is saphenofemoral or saphenopopliteal incompetence or both. Always palpate lower limb pulses in patients with varicose veins. This is especially important if surgery is contemplated.

Tap test

The saphenofemoral junction is one finger's breadth below and lateral to the pubic tubercle. Make the patient cough looking towards the opposite side with your fingers over the saphenofemoral junction. A transmitted impulse to the fingers denotes an incompetent saphenofemoral junction. Tap the saphenofemoral junction whilst feeling lightly over the varicosities over the thigh or below the knee. A transmitted impulse to these varicosities indicates that a continuous column of blood exists from the saphenofemoral junction to these varicosities as well as incompetence of the valves in between. Normally functioning valves in the long saphenous vein are unidirectional, allowing blood to flow from periphery towards the heart, but not in the reverse direction.

A similar tap test can be carried out over the saphenopopliteal junction whilst lightly palpating the varicosities on the lateral and posterolateral aspect of the calf for a transmitted impulse at the same time. This test helps map the exact territory of individual varicose clusters.

Ask the patient regarding any episodes of thrombophlebitis and carefully palpate the affected area. Gauge its distance from saphenofemoral or the saphenopopliteal junction. Thrombophlebitis ascending to the groin or the knee crease requires urgent duplex as there is the potential danger for pulmonary embolism by escape of clot into the deep venous system.

Examine the quality of skin over any varicosities that are unduly prominent and assess the potential for ulceration and haemorrhage especially around the ankle.

Compare the girth of both thighs and calves. Patients with gross superficial venous incompetence or combined deep and superficial venous incompetence often have an appreciable increase in the girth of the affected calf. An increased calf and thigh girth with typical skin changes in the gaiter area and florid superficial varicosities may indicate underlying gross deep venous incompetence or deep venous obstruction. This is the aftermath of variable amounts of recanalization

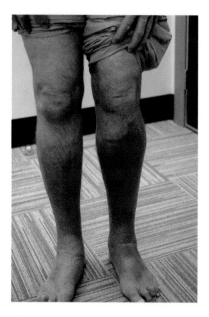

Figure 8.39.   A post-phlebitic limb. Note oedema and pigmentation over left leg.

of the deep veins following an episode/episodes of deep venous thrombosis. This condition is commonly known as a **post-phlebitic limb**.

A tourniquet test known as Perthe's test is useful as a field test to test for deep venous obstruction or deep venous and perforator incompetence in the post-phlebitic limb. A rubber phlebology tourniquet is tied around the mid-thigh area, tight enough to occlude the superficial venous system with the patient prone and his leg raised to collapse all superficial veins; the patient then stands up. Quick refilling of varicosities below the tourniquet on standing up indicates saphenopopliteal incompetence if varicosities are predominantly lateral or posterolateral in distribution. Quick refilling of varicosities over the medial or posteromedial aspect indicates gross perforator incompetence. The patient then walks quickly for 100 to 200 yards. Bulging varicosities indicate perforator incompetence associated with deep venous incompetence. Bursting pain in the calf and bulging varicosities indicates underlying deep venous obstruction. Thus superficial varicosities in patient's with underlying deep venous obstruction are merely bypass vessels and stripping or avulsion of these may only worsen the patient's symptoms. This test cannot, however, replace the accuracy and reproducibility of duplex ultrasound.

Examine the skin over the gaiter area. This is the circumferential area just above the malleoli over the lower third of the calf. Look for signs of venous hypertension. These include localised eczema, brownish pigmentation due to the breakdown of extravasated red blood cells and dermatitis due to the breakdown products of haem. There is atrophy of subcutaneous fat and fibrosis (lipodermatosclerosis). This is the result of local hypoxia as a result of pericapillary "cuffing" due to extravasation of fibrin and other plasma proteins. This extravasation of red blood cells and plasma proteins is the result of increased hydrostatic pressure in capillaries, a direct reflection of severe venous hypertension at the ankle (80–90 mmHg) as a result of gravity and valvular incompetence. Lipo-dermatosclerosis precedes venous ulceration.

Aways examine the groin and lower limb for any signs of previous surgery for varicose veins.

Various types of intricate tourniquet tests have been devised to look for associated deep venous obstruction, perforator incompetence and to determine the level of incompetence. These tests are unreliable and mostly inconclusive. They take unnecessary time and are uncomfortable for the patient and clinician. Therefore, these have been replaced entirely by venous duplex.

Examination of Venous Ulcer

Venous ulcers develop over the medial or lateral aspect of the gaiter area depending on whether there is incompetence in the saphenofemoral or the saphenopopliteal territory, respectively. These patients are more likely to have associated perforator incompetence and deep venous incompetence. These ulcers are shallow, painful and frequently infected. There is a profuse exudate and it is not uncommon to have colonisation with pseudomonas. There is accompanying greenish tinge

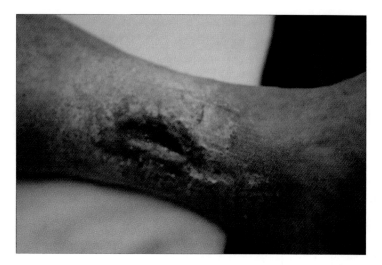

Figure 8.40.   Venous ulcer.

and distinctive odour in these cases. There is surrounding pigmentation and an area of lipodermatosclerosis, giving a brawny indurated feel to the surrounding area. With time, ulceration surrounds the gaiter area in a circumferential manner and the episodes of partial healing and accompanying fibrosis followed by outbreaks of ulcers leads to an inverted champagne bottle appearance.

Older patients may have coexisting arterial insufficiency and careful palpation of pulses is essential. Frequently, an ankle-brachial pressure index is impractical due to a painful ulcer at the ankle and in this situation, toe pressure or a toe-brachial pressure index is most useful in estimating vascular reserve and planning further intervention.

Recurrent cellulitis and lymphangitis around a longstanding venous ulcer leads to damage and fibrosis of lymphatic vessels. This eventually leads to lymphoedema. Previous varicose vein surgery especially redo surgery may exacerbate lymphoedema as lymph nodes and lymphatic channels may already be compromised by this.

Thus, it is not uncommon to have brawny non-pitting oedema in patients with long-standing venous ulceration. This lymphoedema may add to the girth of a post-phlebitic limb.

Examination of Lymphoedema

Lymphoedema is an accumulation of protein-rich tissue fluid in the extracellular compartment as a result of defective lymphatic function. There is sequestration of lymphocytes, monocytes and Langerhans cells in this fluid. Production of cytokines results in proliferation of fibroblast and epithelial cells causing sclerotic changes in skin and subcutaneous tissues. The incidence of lymphoedema is three times higher in females.

Lymphoedema may be primary (unknown cause) or secondary to damage to lymphatics by a known pathologic process.

Patients who present early have pitting oedema with normal skin texture. Later, with subcutaneous fibrosis, the oedema is non-pitting.

Later, skin becomes rough, dry and verrucous. Some patients develop vesicles and these leak chyle. There is maceration and secondary infection with yeasts and fungi.

Recurrent episodes of lymphangitis and cellulitis lead to worsening of lymphoedema.

Points to note in the history are: travel to the tropics, history of any cancer surgery, such as an inguinal lymph node dissection or an axillary clearance. A history of radiotherapy to the chest or the pelvis is also relevant. A careful examination of the affected extremity with regard to skin lesions, such as a melanoma is important. Examination of the draining lymph nodes as well as lymph nodes elsewhere is also important. An examination of the chest and abdomen will help rule out any axial masses associated with the lymphoedema.

Secondary lymphoedema can also occur after longstanding venous ulceration, due to recurrent cellulitis and lymphangitis.

Patient with lymphoedema over left leg after excision of a melanoma and en-bloc excision of inguinal lymph nodes.

Primary Lymphoedema

More than one-third of these patients have a family history of lymphoedema. Usually, the lower limb is affected. Sometimes the scrotum, face or genitalia are affected. Upper limbs are affected very rarely.

Congenital Lymphoedema

True congenital lymphoedema is hereditary and presents within one year of birth. This is the result of hypoplasia or aplasia of lymphatics and affects males more than females.

Some patients with congenital lymphoedema have lymphatic hyperplasia with poorly functioning lymphatic channels.

Megalymphatics

Affect boys and girls equally and may be associated with leak into the abdomen, pleural cavity or the urinary tract. These patients have absent lymphatic valves, thus leading to a reflux of lymph under the influence of gravity. Skin vesicles are common and these leak chyle.

Late onset primary oedema

This is more common than congenital lymphoedema. Women are affected more than men. These can be divided into two groups:

- Distal obliterative lymphoedema: The proximal lymphatic channels may be unaffected and in these patients the swelling is confined to below the knee. This condition becomes apparent around puberty.
- Proximal obliterative lymphoedema: These patients presents at any age after puberty. The swelling initially affects the thigh but then eventually progresses to involve the whole limb. These patients have fibrosed inguinal and pelvic lymph nodes. Initially the lymphatics in the distal part of the limb are dilated and then eventually fibrose and reduce in number.

Secondary Lymphoedema

These have varied causes:

- Filariasis due to *Wuchereria bancrofti*, *Brugia malayi* and *Brugia timori* are caused by transmission of these parasites by various arthropod vectors. These parasites enter the lymphatics and cause a inflammatory process in the lymph nodes.

- Non-filarial elephantiasis in tribesman from East Africa and Ethiopia caused by an obstructive lymphopathy as a reaction to silicates absorbed from soil by walking barefoot.
- Chronic infections such as tuberculosis, hidradenitis suppurativa and lymphogranuloma venereum.
- Recurrent acute bacterial infections in lower limbs in patients with chronic wounds such as venous ulcers.
- Lymph node dissection, open vascular reconstructive surgery or lymph node clearance.
- Primary or secondary malignancy in lymph nodes.
- Radiotherapy causing lymphatic fibrosis.

Lymphangiosarcoma

A rare but fatal complication seen in patients with chronic upper limb lymphoedema following axillary clearance and radiotherapy for breast cancer.

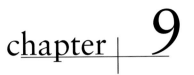
Endocrine Examination

Shamasunder H. Acharya

Introduction

In this chapter we will discuss the important aspects of physical examination of some common endocrine problems, even though they are described in other chapters.

Diabetes Mellitus

CASE STUDY 9.1

A 58-year-old male was referred to the outpatient clinic for management of his type 2 diabetes that was diagnosed five years ago. His current glycaemic control is poor with an HbA1c of 11% and he is also noted to be hypertensive by his family doctor.

History: Ask about primary symptoms of diabetes such as thirst, polyuria, nocturia, and weight loss. Unstable glycaemia may result in blurring of vision and thrush. Profound weight loss is more common in type 1 diabetes but can also occur in poorly controlled type 2 diabetes. Tiredness is also a common symptom of poor glycaemia.

> **Kichu's thoughts . . .**
>
> A patient with diabetes should look after his feet better than his face!

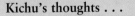

Ask about any claudication pain, angina, previous history of vascular events such as stroke, myocardial infarction and investigations undertaken. Tingling or numbness across the feet together with burning sensation indicates peripheral neuropathy. Erectile dysfunction in males indicates autonomic neuropathy. Diabetic retinopathy may be silent or patients may present with reduced vision due to complications arising from retinopathy.

A detailed family history (diabetes, IHD, autoimmune conditions) should be taken. Note smoking and alcohol intake.

Initial assessment should also include dietary habits with particular attention to refined carbohydrate intake. Note all relevant medications including previous medications that have been discontinued.

Examination: Body mass index (BMI) is usually elevated in patients with type 2 diabetes. A high waist circumference (for example, > 94 cm for men, 80 cm for women) is a measure of abdominal fat and predicts increased cardiovascular risk. Look for acanthosis nigricans, black velvety areas of hyperpigmentation affecting neck, axilla and skin creases. Its presence indicates insulin resistance.

In absence of significant risk factors for type 2 diabetes such as a strong family history or obesity, clinicians should look for any pointers towards secondary diabetes. For example, history of heavy alcohol intake and stigma of chronic liver disease may suggest chronic pancreatitis as a cause of diabetes. Excessive generalised pigmentation with hepatomegaly may be due to haemochromatosis. Acromegalic or cushingoid appearance should prompt the clinician to investigate further. Lipodystrophy syndromes may be associated with insulin resistance and type 2 diabetes.

Take blood pressure and complete general physical examination. Note any features of hyperlipidaemia such as tendon xanthomas. Arcus senilis is common in patients with diabetes.

Feet examination: General observation should include the shape of the feet, hygiene, nails for evidence of fungal infection and callous on the plantar surface. Look for any signs of early vascular insufficiency such as loss of hair. Dryness of skin indicates autonomic neuropathy. Similarly, wasting of small muscles of the feet, clawed toes and prominent metatarsal heads suggest motor neuropathy which predisposes to callus and subsequent ulcers on pressure areas. Note any ulcers, bony deformity and previous amputations.

Check peripheral pulses on dorsalis pedis and posterior tibial arteries. Feel for femoral artery pulses. Note any temperature differences across the feet. A warm, swollen joint could be due to infection or Charcot's joint.

Conduct sensory examination with a 10 g monofilament on at least five different places on the plantar surface of the feet including under the great toe. Test for vibration sense and ankle reflexes. Reduced sensation usually indicates peripheral neuropathy and such patients are considered to be high risk for foot ulcers.

If an ulcer is present, note the size, shape and position of the ulcer. Neuropathic ulcers classically occur on pressure points such as heel or metatarsal heads. Note any malodour from the ulcer and look for signs of infection at the ulcer base and surrounding areas. If bone is visible, osteomyelitis is present. Ischaemic ulcers on the other hand tend to occur on toes and may appear gangrenous. In practice, neuroischaemic ulcers are more common than pure neuropathic or ischaemic ones. Finally, no foot examination is complete, until you have examined the footwear! Ill fitting shoe is often a common precipitant for neuropathic ulcer.

Examine the visual acuity. Note any cataracts. Perform fundoscopy on both eyes looking for any evidence of retinopathy.

Background retinopathy: Microaneurysms, blot haemorrhages and hard exudates.

Pre-proliferative retinopathy: Soft exudates, cotton wool spots, venous abnormalities.

Proliferative retinopathy: Features of background retinopathy with new blood vessels at disc (new vessels appear purposeless and bushy) or elsewhere. Observe any retinal haemorrhage, evidence of previous laser therapy.

Look at the fovea (easier if you ask the patient to look at the light) and look for exudates around the macula (maculopathy).

Assess the patient for autonomic neuropathy when relevant.

Assessment of a Patient with Type I Diabetes

Routine assessment should include examination of the feet, BP and fundoscopy at least annually. Assess glycaemic control by going through home glucose monitoring results, frequency and severity of hypoglycaemia. Frequent hypoglycaemia may result in loss of warning, which has implications on driving and occupation. Ask patients routinely about hypoglycaemia awareness.

Necrobiosis lipoidica is an inflammatory skin condition commonly seen in young women with poorly controlled type 1 diabetes. Look for oval shaped lesions with reddish brown edges and yellowish centre which may be ulcerated. Tiny blood vessels are sometimes seen at the edges. Diabetic stiff joint syndrome is due to tight waxy skin and joint rigidity. Patients are unable to approximate palms together as in prayer sign.

Postural hypotension, inadequate pupillary responses to light, symptoms of gastroparesis such as nausea, vomiting, dysphagia, bowel disturbance and gustatory sweating indicates autonomic neuropathy. This can be confirmed by checking postural systolic BP drop of > 30 mmHg and loss of sinus arrhythmia (ask the patient to take deep inspiration and expiration for 5 s while attached to ECG tracings; < 10 beat/min variation is abnormal).

Look for evidence of co-existing autoimmune conditions such as vitiligo, Addison's disease or Graves' disease.

Examination of the injection sites may reveal areas of lipohypertrophy, which can cause unreliable insulin absorption and erratic glucose control.

Examination of the Thyroid

CASE STUDY 9.2

A 22-year-old lady presents to you with a three-month history of weight loss and palpitations. She has also noticed a lump in her neck.

History: Patients with hyperthyroidism usually describe heat intolerance, excessive sweating, palpitations, weight loss despite a good appetite, insomnia and increased frequency of bowel movements. In addition to this, ask for any pressure symptoms associated with enlarged thyroid such as dysphagia, dysphonia and dyspnoea.

Enquire about any eye symptoms such as grittiness, discomfort, redness, pain or visual disturbance which may be due to Graves' ophthalmopathy. Severe cases present with reduced vision, altered colour vision and corneal ulcer. Urgent ophthalmological assessment is necessary to save vision.

Past medical history of thyroid illness, medications such as amiodarone or iodine preparations and radiation exposure should be elicited. Family history of thyroid dysfunction or any other autoimmune conditions point towards autoimmune aetiology.

Thyroid nodules may be asymptomatic or may present with pain if recently bled. A rapidly enlarging goiter should be investigated for thyroid malignancy.

Examination: Thyroid is best examined while the patient is seated. A restless, anxious fidgety patient usually has severe hyperthyroidism. Note warm and moist hands in hyperthyroidism as opposed to cold and clammy hands in anxiety. Ask the patient to hold his/her hands stretched and observe fine tremors. Check the pulse for tachycardia and rhythm.

Inspect the thyroid gland for any enlargement and observe the thyroid moving upwards while swallowing (ask the patient to drink water). A large goiter may be associated with inspiratory stridor due to compression of trachea. Look for any scars from previous surgery. Note any signs of thyroid eye disease such as exophthalmus, ophthalmoplegia and redness in the eye.

Palpation of thyroid is best done while standing behind the patient. Palpate the thyroid with your fingertips taking care not to cause any discomfort to the patient. You will feel the isthmus of thyroid below cricoid cartilage and over trachea, and two lobes of thyroid extending laterally behind the sternomastoid. Normally the thyroid is barely palpable.

Ask the patient to take a mouthful of water and swallow while you are appreciating the thyroid gland in your fingertips. Note any enlargement, nodularity, consistency or tenderness. Palpate the trachea to see any displacement. Feel for any enlarged lymph nodes in the neck. Percussion on the sternum for retrosternal extension has been traditionally done but has poor predictive value. Auscultate on the enlarged thyroid to hear any bruit associated with increased vascularity in Graves' disease.

A smooth uniform enlargement of thyroid suggests Graves' disease and diagnosis is confirmed on clinical examination alone if thyroid eye disease is present. A nodular enlargement in a hyperthyroid patient suggests the diagnosis of toxic multinodular goiter.

A hard, fixed thyroid is likely to be due to malignancy or Riedel's thyroiditis. Viral thyroiditis usually presents with a very painful thyroid swelling which is firm to hard in consistency.

Confirm the patient is in sinus rhythm and not in cardiac failure.

Extrathyroidal Manifestations of Graves' Disease

Graves' ophthalmopathy (thyroid eye disease)

Retraction of eyelids is very common in hyperthyroidism. Normally eyelids rest 2 mm below the superior limbus and if sclera is visible above the limbus, retraction is present. Similarly, sclera may be visible below the inferior limbus. Ask the patient to look at your finger and follow it downwards. Retraction becomes more obvious.

Proptosis (protrusion of eyeballs) is due to swelling of extraocular muscles and is easier to detect when the patient is seated and examined from above. Proptosis can be unilateral or bilateral. Proptosis is best examined by Hertel exophthalmometer.

Ask the patient to close their eyelids and look for any incomplete closure which may predispose to keratitis or corneal ulcers. Examine the conjunctiva for congestion and oedema.

Check for movements of the eye for double vision which could be due to extraocular muscle involvement.

Check for visual acuity and colour vision with Ishihara colour vision charts. If visual acuity is less than 6/18 or colour vision is affected, urgent ophthalmology referral is indicated. Perform fundoscopy and look for any signs for papilloedema due to severe proptosis or pale discs with optic neuropathy.

Dermopathy (pretibial myxoedema) usually appears as a raised, indurated and discoloured lesion on the shin, dorsum of the feet and rarely on other areas due to accumulation of glycosaminoglycans.

Acropachy is very rare and occurs typically with ophthalmopathy. It presents as clubbing of the digits and is usually painless.

Hypothyroidism

Typically patients present with weight gain, hoarseness of voice, lethargy and cold intolerance. Mild forms are more common than florid forms. Clinical signs would include dull expressionless face, sparse hair, periorbital puffiness, macroglossia and pale cool skin that feels doughy. Look for any previous thyroidectomy scar. Test ankle or supinator jerks and observe the delayed relaxation phase (typically reflexes are not absent but relaxation is delayed). Patients may be hypothermic and bradycardic.

In summary, when examining the patients for thyroid problem, determine the nature of thyroid enlargement, clinical status of the patient (euthyroid, hyperthyroid, hypothyroid), any extrathyroidal signs. Patients may be hyper-, hypo- or euthyroid when they present with goiter. Enquire about any thyroid medication they may have taken.

General Endocrine Examination

History should focus on presenting symptoms; however, symptoms are often non-specific in endocrinology. The following list of symptoms is commonly encountered in endocrinology but it is by no means exhaustive.

- Excessive sweating (hyperthyroidism, acromegaly, anxiety neurosis, constitutional, pheochromocytoma)
- Weight gain (hypothyroidism, Cushing's, obesity)

- Weight loss (hyperthyroidism, poorly controlled diabetes, Addison's disease, Coeliac disease)
- Hirsutism (polycystic ovarian syndrome, Cushing's, racial, adrenal and ovarian neoplasm in women, acromegaly)
- Tiredness (Addison's disease, hypothyroidism, poorly controlled diabetes, hypercalcaemia, Coeliac disease)
- Excessive thirst, polyuria, nocturia (diabetes mellitus or insipidus, hypercalcaemia, psychogenic)
- Increasing hand size, oily skin (acromegaly)
- Poor libido, fatigue, poor muscle strength in men (hypogonadism)
- Galactorrhoea (prolactinoma, hypothyroidism, PCOS, nipple stimulation in addition to physiological causes)
- Flushing (carcinoid syndrome, pheochromocytoma)
- Excessive pigmentation (Addison's disease, ectopic ACTH producing tumours, haemochromatosis)
- Amenorrhoea (primary — Turners' syndrome, uterine agenesis, prolactinoma, constitutional delay, PCOS)
- Amenorrhoea (secondary — prolactinoma, PCOS, anorexia nervosa, hyperthyroidism)
- Spontaneous hypoglycaemia (drugs, insulinoma, Addison's disease, hypopituitarism, sarcomas)
- Gynaecomastia (hypogonadism, drugs, prolactinoma, liver disorder, drugs, testicular tumours)
- Hypopituitarism: Observe pale and smooth skin. Often patients look much younger. Look for visual fields (typically bitemporal hemianopia), optic atrophy on fundoscopy.
- Evidence of previous surgery (transcranial).

Acromegaly

Large hands and feet may be obvious on inspection. Look for coarse facial features and oily skin, enlarged nose, deep nasolabial furrows, prognathism and interdental separation. Increasing skin tags are also common in acromegaly. Patients have deep voice. Check for hypertension, carpel tunnel syndrome and visual field deficits.

Cushing's syndrome

Patients have round face and thin skin with easy bruising. Weight gain is usually central with sparing of limbs which gives rise to "lemon on stick" appearance. Pink abdominal striae, hirsutism, buffalo hump (increased fat pad below the neck posteriorly) and hypertension are some of the features. Test the muscle strength in hip flexors for proximal myopathy. In advanced cases, patient may have had osteoporotic fractures and may complain of reduced height, kyphoscoliosis, etc.

Addison's disease

Patients usually appear thin and excessively pigmented. In less obvious cases, pigmentation should be specifically looked in areas such as skin creases, buccal mucosa and scars. Patients have postural hypotension and may be mildly tachycardic. Secondary sexual hair growth may be reduced or absent in women with Addison's disease.

Male hypogonadism

Skin is usually smooth. Look for bare chest and reduced facial hair growth and secondary sexual hair. Patients may have gynaecomastia (should be differentiated with lipomastia by palpating the breast tissue behind the nipple. Press the nipple and look for any milky discharge). Examine the testicles and external genitalia. Testicles usually measure 20–25 ml in size (check with orchidometer). Small, pea-sized testicles in an adult indicate Klinefelter's syndrome. Similarly, soft and smaller testicles may indicate testicular failure.

Hirsutism

A gradual onset of male pattern hair growth (on face, chest, abdomen and limbs) and menstrual irregularity in a young woman is likely to be due to PCOS but rapid onset of hirsutism, especially in an older woman, may be due to androgen-producing tumours from adrenal or ovary gland. Look for excessive hair growth in chin, over lips, on chest, abdomen and limbs. Ferriman–Gallwey scores assess the severity and the extent of hirsutism. In addition, note any frontal balding, deep voice, increased muscle mass and cliteromegaly when relevant. Note any acanthosis.

Further Reading

Turner H, Wass J. 2002 *Oxford Handbook of Endocrinology and Diabetes.* Oxford University Press: USA.

chapter 10

Examination of the Elderly Patient

Rowan McIlhagger

Introduction

All elderly people are different. Some have complex past medical histories and multiple comorbid conditions, others have had good prior health, even when presenting in their eighties or nineties. Their presenting history may be vague or non-specific, and the physical examination is therefore often of proportionately more importance to the overall clinical assessment.

The approach to the physical examination of the older patient is determined by the patient's past history and current comorbidities, the presenting problem or problems, the purpose of the assessment and

> **Kichu's thoughts . . .**
>
> Remember, if the patient has multiple problems, it is a golden opportunity to intervene at multiple sites.

the setting of the assessment. The more robust older person with a specific single symptom such as chest pain can be approached in an identical manner to the younger patient. The frailer patient with a vaguer presentation such as "off legs" or multiple presenting symptoms will need a different, tailored approach.

Clinical assessment in an acute situation will focus on key areas of relevance to the immediate presentation, whereas assessment in an outpatient or other non-acute setting may permit more comprehensive examination.

The physical examination of the elderly patient presents a number of challenges. These include obstacles to full compliance with examination such as visual or hearing impairment, poor mobility, pain, dysphasia, cognitive impairment and agitation, perhaps secondary to delirium. Multimorbidity is extremely common and multiple physical signs, many of which may not be related to the patient's current problems, are often found. Polypharmacy is also common in older patients, and drugs can cause some signs such as tremor, dry tongue and postural hypotension. These issues are summarised in Table 10.1.

Table 10.1. Implications of old age on the conduct of the physical examination and physical findings as well as their interpretation.

Conduct of the examination	Time	Allow more! It may take longer because of mobility, dependence on others for activities of daily living (e.g. undressing), understanding, compliance and multiple findings.
	Positioning	Flexion contractures, intolerance of lying flat or hemiparesis may make standard positioning difficult.
	Compliance	Patient compliance may be poorer due to communication difficulties or cognitive impairment. Seek help from a nurse or carer.
	Screening	Consider the benefit of routine assessment for common comorbidities that may be undiagnosed (e.g. MMSE for cognitive impairment, rectal examination for prostatic enlargement).
Physical findings and their interpretation	More abnormalities found	Many will be unrelated to the presenting symptom, and reflect comorbidity. Remember that the comorbidity may be previously unrecognised — and may therefore be unaddressed. Document all abnormalities found, whether or not you judge them to be currently relevant.

(Continued)

(Continued)

False positive findings	A sign can be regarded as a false positive if it is present but not caused by the primary pathology of interest. For example, leg oedema has many causes, of which heart failure is one. If you are considering a diagnosis of heart failure after taking the history, the finding of oedema may be due to some other problem, and may be a "false positive" sign for heart failure. Such signs are also described as of low specificity.
False negative findings	Older patients sometimes don't display a sign that is expected to be found in association with their prime pathology or problem. For example, tachycardia may not occur or be less pronounced in association with volume depletion. This can be considered as a "false negative" finding.
Drug treatment	Drug treatment is common in older patients and may make some signs less prominent (e.g. tachycardia in GI haemorrhage in a patient on a beta adrenoreceptor blocker) or be the cause of the sign (e.g. chorea in a patient on antiparkinsonian medication).

Given the non-specific nature of the presentation of illness in the old and the need to always look for treatable problems, no matter how simple, even in the frailest old, positive findings on physical examination should always be regarded as potential indicators of underlying disease, rather than due to age alone.

This chapter suggests an approach to the clinical examination and interpretation of physical findings of older people, as well as highlights commonly encountered differences.

It will give practical advice on carrying out the physical examination, highlight key areas of examination that are particularly relevant to the elderly patient, and use a problem-based approach to enable the reader to perform a focused but thorough examination when faced with common conditions presenting in the elderly.

Conducting the Examination

A number of general points should be considered when examining an elderly person. These serve to assist both doctor and patient by allowing as thorough an assessment as possible, whilst maintaining high standards of comfort and dignity for the patient.

Environment

The examination should ideally take place in a warm, quiet, well-lit room that is free from distractions. Physical assessment of older patients invariably takes a little longer — always allow for extra time particularly if a comprehensive examination is required.

Personnel

It is often helpful to have a nurse or care assistant present to help with the transferring, positioning and undressing of the patient. They can also act as a chaperone if appropriate.

Consent and Understanding

Sensory and/or cognitive impairment can make it difficult to obtain consent from an elderly person. The doctor should always be satisfied that the patient, or, if they lack the capacity to consent, their next of kin, has consented before carrying out the examination. Always explain what you are planning to do, both before you start and as you proceed through the examination. The more the patient understands, the more likely it is that they will be able to comply with the examination and help you to help them.

Sensory Impairment

Many elderly people suffer from visual and/or hearing loss, and this can be an obstacle to effective examination. This may be addressed by simple measures such as ensuring the patient is wearing their spectacles or hearing aids. In patients with profound hearing loss, communicator devices can be useful, as can written instructions.

Cognitive Impairment

The impact of cognitive impairment on clinical examination is very variable, and depends on the degree of cognitive impairment, as well as the presence or absence of agitation or altered awareness or arousal, as may be the case in delirium. The approach required will depend on the circumstances, but in general, clear, one-stage commands give the patient the best chance of being able to comply. In the agitated patient, examination may have to be done in an opportunistic rather than a systematic way. For example, if the patient leans forward for some reason this will allow a quick auscultation of the lung bases. The doctor should be prepared to adapt their routine to meet the needs of the patient, rather than expecting the patient to comply with the doctor's routine.

Integrating the Examination

Physical examination is sometimes focused on specific areas of relevance to a presenting complaint (e.g. the respiratory and cardiovascular systems in a patient with breathlessness) and sometimes comprehensive and systematic (e.g. in a patient with multiple symptoms or vague general decline). Clinicians should always consider how to integrate their examination routine in a way that minimises movement for the patient and maximises their understanding and cooperation (Skrastins *et al.*, 1982). Compliance will, in general, be better if the clinician explains what they are about to do and why they are doing it in simple terms.

A General Approach to Examining Elderly Patients

The detailed approach to physical examination of each system is covered in the relevant chapters of this book. This section highlights potential areas of difficulty that may be encountered when undertaking the general examination, and examination of each of the major systems in older patients.

Vital signs

The haemodynamic response to acute illness may be modified by comorbidity, frailty or drug treatment. Autonomic and baroreceptor dysfunction becomes increasingly prevalent and the heart rate response to sepsis or hypovolaemia may also be blunted. Concurrent use of medications, particularly beta adrenoreceptor blockers, may also blunt the heart rate response to acute illness. Temperature response to infection may be reduced (Norman *et al.*, 1985) and significant focal infection, bacteraemia or sepsis may all be present without pyrexia. Hypothermia may also occur in sepsis or as a feature of other subacute illness and should be specifically sought if low-reading thermometers are not in routine use.

General appearance

Some older people, particularly those living alone, or with the frailty syndrome (see Table 10.2) or cognitive impairment, may have difficulty maintaining standards of personal hygiene, grooming or appearance. Hair and clothes may be unclean, toenails unkempt and

Table 10.2.   The frailty syndrome.

Diagnose the frailty syndrome if three or more of the following are present:

Unintentional weight loss (10 lb in last year)
Self-reported exhaustion
Weakness (grip strength)
Slow walking speed
Low physical activity

facial hair longer than was the patient's habit in younger life. Note such findings, as they may have relevance to the patient's overall functional status, circumstances, condition and outlook.

Frailty

Recently, the concept of frailty as a distinct clinical syndrome has been developed. Studies have suggested that the presence of a frailty phenotype is an independent predictor of falls, disability and death (Fried *et al.*, 2001; Rockwood *et al.*, 2005). Specific features of the syndrome, as described below should be sought and documented.

Skeletal Deformity

It is important to note the presence and functional impact of any skeletal deformity. Some common examples are shown below.

Nutritional Status

It is very important to assess the nutritional status of elderly patients routinely as subnutrition will suggest the need for dietetic input, pressure area and skin care, and increase morbidity and mortality. Always document a patient's weight on admission and at every clinic

Table 10.3.   Common skeletal deformities in older people.

Sign	Likely pathology	Possible consequences
Kyphosis	Osteoporotic vertebral collapse	Pain, decreased mobility, respiratory compromise
Bowed tibia	Paget's disease	Pain, decreased mobility, falls
Leg shortening and external rotation	Fractured neck of femur	Pain, significant morbidity, death
Joint swelling/ tenderness/ deformity/erythema	Arthritis	Sepsis, pain, decreased mobility, falls, increased dependence

visit. Body mass index (BMI) is a useful measurement and is obtained by dividing a patient's weight in kg by the square of their height in metres. Measurement of arm span or knee height can be used to estimate height when a patient has severe kyphosis or is bedridden (Mitchell *et al.*, 1982). Remember that the presence of significant oedema will increase BMI, and that subtle signs of malnutrition such as thinning of the hair and ecchymoses may be confused with common age-related changes. Loss of orbital fat may cause a sunken appearance to the eyes and so called "senile ptosis".

Inspection of the oral cavity is important, as lack of teeth, poor oral hygiene or ill-fitting dentures will all increase the risk of malnutrition. Signs of specific vitamin or nutrient deficiency such as angular stomatitis or gingivitis may also be present. Inspection of the skin may yield further information, with pallor being suggestive of anaemia resulting from iron or folate deficiency. Evidence of recent weight change such as loose skin folds or striae is likely to be significant, and the presence of excessive bruising may indicate a lack of vitamins C or K.

A variety of chronic diseases, including heart failure, COPD, pulmonary fibrosis and rheumatoid arthritis, can be associated with substantial loss of body weight and contribute to the development of cachexia or the frailty syndrome.

Hydration and Volume Status

Dehydration is common in older patients and associated with a high morbidity and mortality. It can be difficult to detect, and accurate monitoring of intake and output should be a key part of the care of in-patients. The relative effects of the loss of a given volume of water are more significant as total body water is reduced in older age. In other words, having diarrhoea for 24 hours may have a more profound effect on hydration than would be in the case of a younger patient.

Fluid depletion is suggested by decreased skin turgor, hypotension or a postural drop in blood pressure, tachycardia, low JVP and dry mucous membranes. Clinical assessment of dehydration is, however, difficult. Skin turgor is better assessed on the forehead or sternum (Viranti *et al.*, 2007) than the dorsum of the hand given the changes in subcutaneous connective tissue that occur with ageing. A dry mouth can indicate dehydration but it is also a common side effect of many medications taken by elderly people, and can also be caused by oxygen administration and open-mouth breathing. Therefore, dryness of mouth should not be relied upon solely in hydration status assessment (McGee *et al.*, 1999).

A change in the blood pressure from a recently recorded value is often a more valuable indicator than the absolute blood pressure at the time of assessment. The prevalence of systolic hypertension increases with age, so the significance of a systolic pressure of 120 mmHg may be greater in an older patient than a younger patient. Compare current values with previous measurements for more meaningful assessment.

Postural hypotension is also more prevalent with increasing age and is therefore a less specific sign of volume depletion than in younger patients (McGee *et al.*, 1999). Postural tachycardia, conversely, may not be so pronounced in the presence of volume depletion if autonomic dysregulation (or concomitant treatment with beta blockade) is present. Capillary refill time is also prolonged in some older patients, reducing the specificity of this sign for volume depletion (Schriger *et al.*, 1988).

When considering whether the patient is volume overloaded, review the jugular venous pressure and look for oedema, particularly in the lower limbs or sacrum if the patient has been nursed in bed. Both an elevated jugular venous pressure and oedema can however be caused by alternate problems (heart failure and venous insufficiency, respectively) and are not necessarily indicative of volume overload.

Skin Integrity

Studies of hospital and community patients have shown prevalence rates of pressure sores of between 5.3% and 8.8%, with 70% occurring in those aged over 70 years (Young *et al.*, 1992). Estimates of the total cost to the UK NHS range from £150 million in 1982 to £750 million in 1994 (West *et al.*, 1994), and the presence of a pressure sore leads to an increase in relative mortality of up to five times (Young *et al.*, 1992). Broken skin is a potential source of occult sepsis and pain in an unwell patient, and usually requires specialist nursing care; therefore, it is important to make a thorough assessment of pressure areas. The toes and feet should also be inspected carefully, and bandages or dressings removed as soon as practicable to assess the viability and condition of underlying skin, particularly if occult sepsis is a possibility. This should particularly apply to patients with risk factors for skin damage such as poor mobility, wearing of splints or casts, high or low body mass index, long-term corticosteroid use and incontinence.

Pain and Tenderness

Pain is highly prevalent in older people. Patients may however underreport or underemphasize the significance of pain, or present their pain in atypical manners, for example, with relative quietness or withdrawal from usual activities in association with dementia. Seek pain points actively and in specific locations according to the presentation. For example, if sepsis is suspected, seek tenderness in the spine, abdomen and large joints specifically and carefully.

Care should be taken when examining older patients to ensure that unnecessary pain is avoided, particularly when moving the patient around, and examining the extremities, as joint symptoms are common. Fear of pain during examination may be a real barrier to compliance — remember that the last doctor may not have been as careful as you!

Mobility

Poor mobility has major implications for elderly patients, and affects their ability to live independently, as well as increasing their risk of pressure sores, falls and fractures. Information can be gained from observation as the patient enters the consulting room. Note if the patient is walking unaided, with assistance from another person or walking aid, or if they are wheelchair-bound. If using a wheelchair, note if they can self propel. If a walking aid is used, it should be noted if it is the appropriate type and size and if it is being used correctly. The patient's ability to transfer, for example from the chair to the examination couch, can be directly observed. In the history, enquire what assistance is needed within the house, on stairs, in transfers and out of doors. Once identified, mobility disorders should be analysed in a four-stage process.

1. The patient's perspective

Start by asking the patient why they believe that their mobility is poor. Specifically, is their walking worse because of pain (if so, where), weakness (generalised or specific to one limb), poor balance, or low confidence and fear of falling?

2. The neurological examination

Undertake a full neurological examination, particularly, look for physical signs to suggest upper motor neurone disease of the lower limbs (most commonly due to cerebrovascular disease), lower motor neurone disease of the lower limbs (think of lumbar spinal stenosis or peripheral neuropathy), extrapyramidal disease (parkinsonism); proprioceptive disorders and cerebellar disease. Check for Romberg's sign and if the patient has noted dizziness or unsteadiness to be part of the problem; check postural blood pressure and neck movements.

3. The legs

Review the lower limbs in general. Muscle bulk and power may be impaired because of disuse and deconditioning rather than specific neurological disease. Undertake a basic review of the range of movement of each lower limb and the hip, knee and ankle joints. Osteoarthritis, in particular, may cause pain or joint deformity that limits movement and compromise mechanical function. Is the skin of the legs and feet intact? Check the feet for calluses or deformity. Is the footwear appropriate? Is there oedema (leg weight may increase significantly) or evidence of arterial disease (check peripheral pulses) causing pain on exercise or ulceration?

4. Overall function

Undertake a functional gait assessment. What can the patient actually do? Observe them walking — alone, with their walking aids or with another's assistance. Some gait patterns can be recognised but there are often mixed or non-specific findings. Consider recording a specific objective functional gait assessment such as the "timed up and go" test, a reliable and valid test for quantifying functional mobility (Podsiadlo *et al.*, 1991).

The patient is observed and timed while he/she rises from an armchair, walks three metres, turns, walks back, and sits down again. The normal time required to finish the test is between 7 and 10 seconds. Individuals who cannot complete the task in that time probably have mobility problems, especially if they take longer than 20 seconds. More detailed tests such as the Tinetti functional assessment can also provide further information about remediable problems (Tinetti *et al.*, 1986).

Assessment of Mental State

Cognitive assessment is an essential part of the examination of the elderly person, both to diagnose conditions that impair thinking and also as part of the assessment of overall functional ability. One in six people over 80 and one in 14 people over 65 has a form of dementia (http://www.alzheimers.org.uk/downloads/Dementia_UK_Full_Report.pdf). and therefore cognitive assessment should be carried out when examining all elderly people, as previously undiagnosed cognitive impairment may be exposed. Also, impaired cognitive function has an adverse effect on in-hospital mortality (Campbell *et al.*, 2005). Many standardised assessment tools are available (Shulman *et al.*, 2006) but the most commonly used in the UK, US, Australia and Canada is the Mini Mental State Examination (MMSE) (Folstein *et al.*, 1975).

Table 10.4.   Common abnormalities of gait in older people.

Gait	Description	Common causes in the elderly
Parkinsonian	Slow, shuffling, stooped posture, loss of arm swing, "freezing" (e.g. when going through a doorway), difficulty in turning 180°	Idiopathic Parkinson's disease, vascular parkinsonism, Parkinson's plus syndromes
Hemiplegic	One leg stiff, without flexion at knee or ankle, with each step rotated away from the body then towards it, forming a semicircle	Stroke disease
"Cautious gait"	Like walking on ice — slow, short stride length, reduced arm swing, stooped posture	Fear of falling, visual or proprioceptive problems
Ataxic	Broad-based, staggering	Cerebellar/vestibular dysfunction
Antalgic	A limp, in which a phase of the gait is shortened on the injured side to alleviate the pain experienced when bearing weight on that side	Pain from any cause
"Senile gait disorder"	Lower limb parkinsonian type features including shuffling and freezing, sometimes with apraxia and a wide base but little or no upper limb signs	Diffuse cerebrovascular disease
Foot drop	Foot slaps onto floor, patient may accommodate by raising the thigh excessively	Damage to common peroneal nerve or L5 nerve root

This comprises questions testing a variety of cognitive functions including orientation, concentration, recall and calculation. It is quick to perform but it is of limited use in those with hearing or visual impairment, illiteracy or dysphasia. Other factors that may influence the score include language barriers, level of education and premorbid IQ. The Addenbrook's Cognitive Examination takes longer to

Table 10.5.   The Abbreviated Mental Test.

How old are you? (Answer +/– 1 year)
What time is it now? (Answer +/– 1 hour)
What is the name of this place?
Can you remember this address — e.g. 42 West Street? (Ask the patient to recall at end of test)
When did the First World War begin?
What is the Queen's first name?
When is your birthday?
Can you recognise two people?
Can you count down from 20 to 1?
What year is it?

---

perform but includes tests of attention and orientation, memory, fluency, language and visuospatial function. In this test (scored out of 100), a score of less than 88 gives 94% sensitivity and 89% specificity for dementia, and a score of less than 82 gives 84% sensitivity and 100% specificity for dementia (Mioshi *et al.*, 2006). Serial measurements can be used to monitor progress or response to treatment.

In the emergency room situation, such detailed assessment is often impractical, but an Abbreviated Mental Test (scored out of 10) can be quickly undertaken and is a useful screening tool.

Communication

Impairment of the ability to communicate is common, particularly in frailer, older patients. A systematic approach to evaluation is worthwhile — never assume that a poorly communicative patient has dementia, you will miss other important problems.

First note whether the patient responds appropriately to your greeting or introduction. If you think there may be a communication problem, try to decide if you think it is because they can't hear or understand you, or can't express themselves to you, or both.

The problem or problems causing the communication difficulty will be one or more of the "Seven D's".

1. **Deafness**. Is there evidence of hearing impairment? Check hearing formally, find out if the patient can follow written commands.

2. **Dysphasia.** This can be expressive, receptive or mixed. Can the patient name familiar objects, follow simple verbal commands, repeat their name and address?
3. **Dysarthria.** Here the problem is in the formation or articulation of words. Ask the patient to repeat their name and address, note carefully which sounds they have difficulty with. The problem may relate to the tongue, lips or palate. Not uncommonly it will be due to simple problems such as ill-fitting dentures or a dry mouth.
4. **Dysphonia.** The patient hears you, but you find it difficult to hear the patient. Low voice volume may be a feature of many neurological problems including parkinsonism.
5. **Dementia.** Cognitive difficulty may cause slowness or absence of response or difficulty in following commands. Word finding difficulty may also be apparent and it can be difficult to distinguish the problem from dysphasia due to more localised neurological disease.
6. **Delirium.** In addition to cognitive dysfunction, arousal or awareness may be altered and compromise communication.
7. **"Double Dutch".** The patient speaks another language! Find a translator!

Mood

Studies report a wide variety of incidence of depression in the elderly population (Djernes, 2006). However, mood should be assessed in the elderly as depression can often present in an atypical manner, such as weight loss or pseudodementia. Detailed mood questionnaires are usually inappropriate for those with cognitive impairment, and the Geriatric Depression Score (Brink *et al.*, 1982) is commonly used as a screening tool to assess mood. A score of 5–10 out of 15 suggests mild depression, and a score of 11 or more suggests severe depression.

Sensory Loss

Impairments of vision and hearing are highly prevalent, often functionally limiting and frequently improvable.

Hearing loss will often be apparent in the consultation itself, but some patients may not indicate the degree of the problem, leading doctors to assume that the problem is one of cognition rather than hearing. Ask the patient directly about their hearing, and test sound detection simply with voice, finger clicking or paper rustling in each ear. Inspect the ear for wax or abnormality of the drum. Weber and Rinne tests may help decide if the problem is conductive or sensorineural. Familiarise yourself with the basic models of hearing aid used in your locality — learn how to check if they are on or off and to adjust the volume.

Visual difficulty may contribute to poor mobility and falls, limited safety awareness and functional impairment and can lead to social isolation. Ask the patient if they can read the newspaper or see the television. Assess vision in each eye simply by perception of light, hand movement, finger counting or with formal charts, with and without any spectacles. Specifically examine for cataract, macular degeneration and glaucoma. Seek field defects or visual inattention with the appropriate techniques.

Continence

Incontinence is a common problem in the elderly and can have significant implications for independent living, carer stress, skin damage and infections. One study of community-dwelling people over 65 years old found that 31% of women and 23% of men had been incontinent of urine in the past month (Stoddart *et al.*, 2001). This figure is much higher in institutional settings. Clear guidelines about the assessment of urinary incontinence are available (Scottish Intercollegiate Guideline Network, 2004). A full assessment includes a detailed history to elicit risk factors and type of incontinence in women, and prostatic symptoms in men, along with a symptom diary if the patient or carer is able to keep one. Cognitive impairment from any cause may make incontinence more likely and is sometimes the sole explanation. Assessment of a patient with incontinence should therefore include assessment of cognition. Poor mobility may make incontinence more likely to occur (the "shortened wetting distance") but is not commonly the only explanation.

Table 10.6.   Types of prolapse.

Uterovaginal	Uterus into vagina First degree to third degree (complete procidentia)
Cystocele	Bladder into vagina
Enterocele	Small intestine into vagina (finger cannot enter sac on PR exam)
Rectocele	Rectum into vagina (finger can enter sac on PR exam)

Physical Examination of Women

Abdominal examination for a palpable bladder or pelvic masses is required. Although specialist assessment by a gynaecologist may be needed, generalists can undertake a simple examination with a chaperone. The perineum should be inspected for signs of atrophic vaginitis or infection. Stress incontinence can be elicited by asking the patient to cough. A vaginal examination should be performed, looking for prolapse or other abnormalities which would require gynaecological assessment.

Physical Examination of Men

Abdominal examination should be performed, again looking for a palpable bladder. External genitalia should be examined, and a rectal examination performed to assess prostatic size, shape and consistency.

Faecal Incontinence

Assessment of faecal incontinence should include testing of perineal sensation and anal tone, as well as a rectal examination looking for faecal impaction and evidence of overflow incontinence, or a rectal mass. Abdominal examination may reveal evidence of colonic masses, including faecal masses, or distension. Assessment of cognitive function is important, particularly if the patient is incontinent of formed stool.

Examination of the Systems

As discussed above, common dilemmas on systems examination include whether a physical finding is relevant to the patient's current active problems or a sign of an asymptomatic comorbidity, and whether a physical finding is related to age in itself or a specific disease process. In general, it is always best to record all physical findings in case they may prove of relevance to the current or future care of the patient, and to always regard a physical finding as evidence of a disease rather than age alone. Cardiac auscultation provides an example. Systolic murmurs are common in the elderly (Pomerance, 1968), and can often be attributed to aortic sclerosis. Although they increase in prevalence with age they are not ubiquitous, and, as with other physical signs, it is prudent to regard their presence as potentially indicative of relevant disease rather than innocent findings relating to age alone. Clinicians assessing older people should always record detected signs, and attempt to discover whether they are new, old or changing.

> **Kichu's thoughts . . .**
>
> If you cannot get a proper history, think of the "D's".

The full details of individual system examination are covered in other chapters, and this section considers for each major system:

1. The common conditions affecting that system in the elderly.
2. How age may modify clinical signs.
3. How drug treatments may modify clinical signs.

Cardiovascular System

Common conditions affecting the cardiovascular system in the elderly include hypertension, atrial fibrillation, ischaemic heart disease, congestive cardiac failure and valvular heart disease. Murmurs and clinical signs of heart failure are therefore commonly found. "White coat hypertension" also occurs more frequently in the elderly (Niiranen *et al.*, 2006).

Atheromatous vascular disease becomes more prevalent and as such, absence, asymmetry or diminished volume of any peripheral pulse becomes more common. However, these findings or the finding of bruits over carotid, femoral or other major blood vessels should never be regarded as features of normal ageing. A specific form of arterial calcification may be clinically detectable in the radial arteries. This circumferential calcification known as Monckeberg's medial calcification creates a ridged and hardened feeling to the radial artery, traditionally likened to "the trachea of a sparrow". Its presence is weakly associated with systolic hypertension. Auscultation of a fourth heart sound is sometimes regarded by some as a "normal" finding in older age, due to the physiological increase in the atrial contribution to left ventricular filling with age (Spodick *et al.*, 1973). Corneal arcus increases in prevalence in the elderly, but other possible manifestations of dyslipidemia, such as tendon xanthomas, do not. Aortic dilatation may obstruct the left jugular vein, making it an unreliable manometer and giving it a fixed filled appearance. The carotid artery may become more tortuous in its course, making its pulsations easily visible and creating the false impression of arterial dilation, traditionally and somewhat unfairly described as the "student's aneurysm". Kyphosis caused by osteoporotic vertebral collapse can make assessment of the jugular venous pressure difficult, as can the presence of neck or back pain, because positioning the patient optimally may not be possible.

Pulse pressure invariably widens, due predominantly to a rise in systolic arterial pressure. Isolated systolic hypertension (systolic blood pressure over 150 mmHg) becomes more common, but is not an inevitable consequence of ageing. Vascular calcification may artefactually increase the recorded measurement for systolic blood pressure — a phenomenon sometimes described as "pseudohypertension". Although Osler's manoeuvre is suggested to be helpful in determining whether the patient truly has intra-arterial hypertension (Messerli *et al.*, 1985), its practical value has been questioned (Belmin *et al.*, 1995). Systolic and diastolic hypotension are frequent accompaniments of the frailty syndrome and chronic comorbidities such as heart failure and COPD. In frailer patients, such hypotension is said to have adverse prognostic significance.

Several commonly prescribed medications may cause or mask clinical signs in the elderly patient. Beta blockers or rate-limiting calcium channel antagonists may suppress tachycardia in the septic or volume-deplete patient. Conversely, anticholinergics and inhaled or nebulised beta-agonists may lead to a raised heart rate. Many drugs can lead to hypotension or a postural blood pressure drop, the most common of which are antihypertensive agents and diuretics. Some calcium channel blockers may lead to ankle oedema.

Respiratory System

The most common conditions affecting the ageing respiratory system are COPD, interstitial lung disease, bronchiectasis, pneumonia, pulmonary embolus and lung cancer.

An age-related decline in vital capacity has been described and may not be entirely attributable to comorbidity. Chest expansion may be symmetrically reduced, and chest shape abnormalities such as kyphosis secondary to osteoporosis, or hyperinflation secondary to COPD, are more commonly encountered. The presence of crackles (crepitations) is a common finding, but has been shown to be neither a sensitive nor specific indicator of pathology (Connolly et al., 1992). Several conditions such as infection, pulmonary oedema and pulmonary fibrosis can lead to crackles in the chest, and the predominant pathology may be difficult to determine. The systemic effects of prolonged or advanced disease should be remembered — end-stage COPD may cause a cachectic state. Opioid analgesics may alter respiratory rate, and beta adrenoreceptor blockers cause wheeze or prolonged expiration.

Gastrointestinal System

Malnutrition, constipation, faecal incontinence, peptic ulcer disease, malignancy of stomach, colon or pancreas, biliary tract disease, mesenteric ischaemia and diverticular disease are all common conditions in the elderly. On examination, the aorta is often more easily palpable even if it is not enlarged, and care must be taken to assess for the expansile quality that is more likely to indicate aneurysmal dilatation. Kyphosis commonly leads to a transverse abdominal crease, or significant abdominal protrusion, and can also give the impression of apparent hepatomegaly, as the liver is pushed inferiorly. Coexistent hyperinflation of the chest, due perhaps to COPD, may also cause inferior displacement of the liver, detectable by careful percussion of the upper border of the liver. The presence of oedema may mask malnutrition, and oedema or ascites may be due to one or several causes including congestive cardiac failure, low albumin from any cause, and intra-abdominal malignancy. Hepatomegaly may be present in congestive cardiac failure, and may be pulsatile in nature in tricuspid regurgitation. Faecal loading may lead to an apparent abdominal mass, and re-examination following treatment may be necessary to further assess this. Drugs which may modify clinical signs include laxatives which can cause increased activity of bowel sounds and abdominal distension, anticholinergics which can cause a dry mouth, and corticosteroids which, among many other side effects, can lead to an increased body mass index, abdominal striae and bruising.

Neurological System

The most common neurological conditions presenting in the elderly are stroke, cognitive impairment (acute and chronic), parkinsonism and subdural haematoma. Cerebral metastases can also present with neurological symptoms and signs. Common findings on examination are wasting of the small muscles of the hands and general loss of muscle bulk and power, especially at the hips. It is suggested that limitation of upgaze, impairment of vibration sense and mild bradykinesia are the signs most likely to be attributed to age rather than disease. Other signs more commonly observed include the primitive reflexes, sensory loss in the form of reduced smell, taste, increased pain threshold, and, to a lesser extent, proprioception. Physiological tremor may also be observed more frequently.

Table 10.7. Some of the primitive reflexes.

Reflex	Description	Disease
Palmomental	Unilateral contraction of the mentalis and orbicularis oris triggered by brisk scratching of the ipsilateral palm	Alzheimer's
Snout	Pouting or pursing of the lips that is elicited by light tapping of the closed lips near the midline	Disorders affecting frontal lobes, e.g. dementias
Gegenhalten	Involuntary resistance to passive movement	Diffuse forebrain dysfunction, e.g. vascular parkinsonism
Glabellar tap	Continued blinking on repeated taps to the glabella	Extrapyramidal disorders, e.g. Parkinson's disease
Grasp	An involuntary bending of the fingers in response to tactile or tendon stimulation on the palm, producing an uncontrollable grasp	Contralateral frontal lobe damage

Uncertainty has existed about the significance of many of these findings but recent evidence suggests that many neurological signs can be attributed to the neurodegenerative syndromes that accompany ageing rather than ageing per se (Waite *et al.*, 1996). The significance of the absence of ankle reflexes has been a particular area of debate, but the long held view that absent ankle jerks are more common in old age is now contested (Impallomeni *et al.*, 1984),

> **Kichu's thoughts ...**
>
> In my view, the common cause of absent ankle jerk is "poor technique".

as is the true significance of their absence (Bowditch *et al.*, 1996). As a general rule, absence of any deep tendon reflex should be taken to indicate possible disease rather than being dismissed as a feature of age alone. Reflexes may also be harder to elicit in some older people because of arthritis of the lower limbs and consequent difficulty in limb positioning or relaxation. Drugs affecting the neurological system include beta agonists which can cause tremor and antiparkinsonian and antipsychotic medication which can cause chorea and dystonias.

Table 10.8. Common presentations and key signs.

Problem	CVS	RS	GI	Other
Poor mobility	Weak peripheral pulses (claudication) Leg ulcers Leg oedema Signs of heart failure	Signs of COPD	Obesity/cachexia	Loss of muscle mass Focal neurological signs (e.g suggesting stroke/parkinsonism/neuropathy) Bunions/callouses/overgrown toenails Skeletal deformity Pain Cognitive impairment
Acute confusion or agitation	Blood pressure Heart rate Murmurs (infective endocarditis)	Focal signs of consolidation	Abdominal tenderness Faecal loading Palpable bladder Signs of chronic liver disease	Skin turgor Cyanosis Dysphasia/dysarthria Visual field disturbance Focal weakness/neglect/sensory loss Flapping tremor Skin wounds/infection Warm/swollen joints Neck stiffness
Falls/blackouts	Heart rate/rhythm Postural blood pressure Murmur (ESM)			Arthropathy Focal weakness/sensory loss Muscle wasting Injury Bruising Fracture Skin necrosis

(Continued)

(*Continued*)

Problem	CVS	RS	GI	Other
Weight loss	Evidence of heart failure	Evidence of chronic respiratory disease e.g barrel chest	Abdominal mass Organomegaly PR mass (rectum/ prostate)	Poor dentition Clubbing, pallor Breast mass Lymphadenopathy Horner's Fasciculation/wasting Goitre/tremor
Incontinence	Signs of CCF (diuretics may → incontinence)	Signs of COPD/other lung disease → immobility, or cough → stress incontinence	Palpable bladder Rectal impaction Obesity Prostatic enlargement Prolapse Vaginal atrophy	Signs consistent with spinal stenosis/ cord compression Signs consistent with stroke disease/PD/ dementia Arthropathy/neuropathy Cognitive impairment Poor mobility

A Problem Based Approach to Examination

Patients present with problems and not diseases. Their problems may be caused by disease of one, or more frequently several, systems. A comprehensive examination is always preferred, but not always practical, and clinicians should develop an approach to the key examination elements relevant to different presentations. The next table shows some common presentations in the elderly and suggests key signs that should be particularly sought in each case. The list is not exhaustive but should provoke the reader to consider their own approach to a patient presenting with each symptom complex.

Conclusion

A thorough examination of an elderly person can be challenging and time consuming. To achieve as complete an assessment as possible, the key priorities are ensuring maximum comfort and dignity for the patient, considering the potential impact of comorbidity and polypharmacy, and assuming positive clinical findings to be pathological as opposed to be a natural part of the ageing process.

References

1. Belmin J, Visintin JM, Salvatore R, Sebban C, Moulias R. Osler's maneuver: Absence of usefulness for the detection of pseudohypertension in an elderly population. *Am J Med* 1995; 98(1): 42–49.
2. Bowditch MG, Sanderson P, Livesey JP. The significance of an absent ankle reflex. *J Bone Joint Surg* 1996; 78-b: 276–279.
3. Brink TL, Yesavage JA, Lum O, Heersema P, Adey MB, Rose TL. Screening tests for geriatric depression. *Clin Gerontol* 1982; 1: 37–44.
4. Campbell SE, Seymour DG, Primrose WR *et al.* A multi-centre European study of factors affecting the discharge destination of older people admitted to hospital: Analysis of in-hospital data from the ACMEplus project. *Age Ageing* 2005; 34: 467–475.
5. Connolly MJ, Crowley JJ, Vestal RE. Clinical significance of crepitations in elderly patients following acute hospital admission: A prospective study. *Age Ageing* 1992; 21(1): 43–48.

6. Djernes JK. Prevalence and predictors of depression in populations of elderly: A review. *Acta Psychiatr Scand* 2006; 113(5): 372–387.
7. Folstein MF, Folstein SE, McHugh PR. "Mini-mental state." A practical method for grading the cognitive state of patients for the clinician. *J Psych Res* 1975; 12(3): 189–198.
8. Fried LP, Tangen CM, Walston J, Newman AB, Hirsch C, Gottdiener J *et al.* Frailty in older adults: Evidence for a phenotype. *J Gerontol Med Sci* 2001; 56: M146–156.
9. http://www.alzheimers.org.uk/downloads/Dementia_UK_Full_Report.pdf.
10. Impallomeni M, Kenny RA, Flynn MD., Kraenzlin M, Pallis CA. The elderly and their ankle jerks. *Lancet* 1984; 1(8378): 670–672.
11. McGee S, Abernethy W, Simel D. Is this patient hypovolaemic? *JAMA* 1999; 281: 1022–1029.
12. Messerli FH, Ventura HO, Amodeo C. Osler's maneuver and pseudohypertension. *N Engl J Med* 1985; 312(24): 1548–1551.
13. Mioshi E, Dawson K, Mitchell J *et al.* The Addenbrooke's Cognitive Examination Revised (ACE-R): A brief cognitive test battery for dementia screening. *Int J Geriatr Psychiatry* 2006; 21(11): 1078–1085.
14. Mitchell CO, Lipschitz DA. Arm length measurement as an alternative to height in nutritional assessment of the elderly. *Parenter Enteral Nutr* 1982; 6: 226–229.
15. Niiranen TJ, Jula AM, Kantola IM, Reunanen A. Prevalence and determinants of isolated clinic hypertension in the Finnish population: The Finn-HOME study. *J Hypertens* 2006; 24: 463.
16. Norman DC, Grahn D, Yoshikawa TT. Fever and aging. *J Am Geriatr Soc* 1985; 33:859–863.
17. Podsiadlo D, Richardson S. The timed "Up & Go": A test of basic functional mobility for frail elderly persons. *J Am Geriatr Soc* 1991; 39(2): 142–148.
18. Pomerance A. Cardiac pathology and systolic murmurs in the elderly. *Br Heart J* 1968; 30: 687–689.
19. Rockwood K. A global clinical measure of fitness and frailty in elderly people. *CMAJ* 2005; 173(5): 489–495.
20. Schriger DL, Baraff L. Defining normal capillary refill. *Ann Emerg Med* 1988; 17: 932–935.
21. Scottish Intercollegiate Guideline Network. Guideline 79: Management of urinary incontinence in primary care. 2004. http://www.sign.ac.uk/guidelines/published/index.html.
22. Shulman KI, Herrmann N, Brodaty H *et al.* IPA survey of brief cognitive screening instruments. *Int Psychogeriatrics* 2006; 18: 281–294.

23. Skrastins R, Merry GM, Rosenberg GM, Schuman JE. Clinical assessment of the elderly patient. *CMAJ* 1982; 127(3): 203–206.
24. Spodick DH, Quarty-Pigott VM. The fourth heart sound as a normal finding in older persons. *New Engl Med* 1973; 288: 140–141.
25. Stoddart H, Donovan J, Whitley E *et al.* Urinary incontinence in older people in the community: A neglected problem? *Br J Gen Pract* 2001; 51(468): 548–552.
26. Tinetti ME. Performance-oriented assessment of mobility problems in elderly patients. *J Am Geriatr Soc* 1986; 34: 119–126.
27. Vivanti A, Harvey K, Ash S, Battistutta D. Clinical assessment of dehydration in older people admitted to hospital. What are the strongest indicators? *Arch Gerontol Geriatr* 2007; 47: 340–355.
28. Waite LM, Broe GA, Creasey H, Grayson D, Edelbrock D, O'Toole B. Neurological signs, aging, and the neurodegenerative syndromes. *Arch Neurol* 1996; 53: 498–502.
29. West P, Priestley J. Money under the mattress. *Health Serv* 1994; 20–22.
30. Young JB, Dobrzanski S. Pressure sores: Epidemiological and current management concepts. *Drugs Ageing* 1992; 2: 42–57.

Index